# NORMAL

## A PLASTIC SURGEON'S LETTER TO HIS DAUGHTERS ABOUT BODY IMAGE

DR POURIA MORADI

MBBS BSC (MED). MRCS (ENG) FRACS (PLAST)

# DEDICATION

To my wife Jodie and my three daughters Rosie, Evie and Tessa.

My parents and brother, Pezh, his wife Brie and their girls (and Zander)

And all my friends across this beautiful planet.

To Rosie, Evie and Tessa…

"just remember, the unexamined life is not worth living".

First published in 2023 by Pouria Moradi



A catalogue entry for this book is available from the National Library of Australia.

ISBN: 978-1-923007-60-4

Book production and text design by Publish Central
Printed in Australia by McPherson's Printing Group

The paper this book is printed on is environmentally friendly.

**Disclaimer**

The material in this publication is of the nature of general comment only, and does not represent professional advice. It is not intended to provide specific guidance for particular circumstances and it should not be relied on as the basis for any decision to take action or not take action on any matter which it covers. Readers should obtain professional advice where appropriate, before making any such decision. To the maximum extent permitted by law, the author and publisher disclaim all responsibility and liability to any person, arising directly or indirectly from any person taking or not taking action based on the information in this publication. Some names included in this book have been fictionalised for privacy.

# CONTENTS

# INTRODUCTION

*"We repair and restore that which Nature has given,*
*but Fortune has taken away. Not so that it please the eye of the beholder, but so that it buoy the spirit of the afflicted."*

*– Gaspare Tagliacozzi (1545–1599), Father of modern-day plastic surgery*

I first got the idea for this book as I watched my eldest daughter Rosie, who was seven at the time, try on different bathing suits to get ready for her school swimming carnival. She seemed so proud of herself and completely unaware of how she looked. I wondered how long this innocence would last, and feared that some day, in the not-to-distant future, my little girl might be critical of her body and her looks. Would she grow up to see extra kilograms on the scale as the reason to start fad dieting or, worse, starve herself?

As a plastic surgeon, I work with women and girls who hate something about their bodies or their appearance. That got me thinking about my conflicting roles as a father of daughters and a plastic surgeon, and how I could teach my daughters to be confident in their own skin. Rosie's swim events were around the same time Kobe Bryant died in a plane crash with his 13-year-old daughter. I was a competitive basketball player growing up, so I follow the sport closely. The tragic accident was all over the news, which reported on how Bryant was a mentor to his four daughters, and an advocate for female athletes.

As a father of three young girls myself, his passing ignited my own *Mamba Mentality* – to "attack what's in front of you with passion and purpose, without fear and doubt, and without an ounce of quit." I saw it as a sign that I too should write a book, and encourage teens to examine the media images and social pressures that blur the lines between ideal and real. I want them to know the facts about their bodies and what's "normal". I want them to know what to expect should they decide to fix something they dislike about their appearance. I also want to give parents the tools to help raise body-positive girls. I began with a letter to my daughters.

Around this same time, an 18-year-old girl, whom I shall call Alice, came to my office with tuberous breasts (a developmental abnormality that I explain in Chapter Three, *Breast wishes*). As you will read in Alice's emotional story, she did everything she could to hide her figure. Her clothes didn't fit right, and she couldn't wear a bra because one breast was an A cup and the other was a DD cup. At her and her mother's request, I did a procedure to even out her breasts. Afterwards, she said "Thank you, Dr. Moradi, for making me feel normal!"

She was not the first patient to say this very same thing to me. The fact is, most female breasts are asymmetrical, and a slight difference in size should not be a cause for concern. But if you have a condition like Alice's, a one-time surgery can give you a lifetime of confidence. I also see many young women who develop extremely large breasts by the age of 14. The medical term for this is gigantomastia, and it can cause painful back and neck problems as well as unwanted attention and teasing. Fortunately, there's a breast reduction procedure that helps with this too.

Whatever it is that makes children, tweens or teens feel ashamed of how they look – be it a large nose, protruding ears, or birthmarks – the relief and joy my patients feel after surgery is one of the most rewarding parts of my profession. Sadly, girls are often judged harshly. And, as studies clearly show, teens with low self-esteem are more likely to engage in high-risk behaviours such as drugs and alcohol, excessive dieting, unprotected sex, and disordered eating. I address all these things in this book. As I tell my daughters, and now you: try your best to tune out the negative noise, and focus instead on making healthy life choices, including education, nutrition, and exercise.

## MY STORY

Education and physical activity have always been an important part of my life. I played basketball and tennis growing up and, like many boys, I dreamed of being a professional athlete. Becoming a doctor was not on my radar. I love sport because it teaches us teamwork, discipline, and how to deal with failure. I was a good player, but not good enough to make it in the big leagues – as they say, Jack of all trades, master of none.

I grew up in Sydney, and contemplated sitting my SATs for a tennis scholarship in America. I even had an agent lined up, and study notes on how to take the SATs. This did not happen, however, as I was fortunate enough to score well in my HSC, the standardised test for admission to Australian universities. My score got me into the only undergraduate medical school program in Sydney at the University of NSW at the age of 18.

I had decided to switch gears to study medicine at UNSW on a Sam Cracknell Sports and Academic Scholarship, and stopped playing tennis, but continued to play basketball on the varsity team, making lifelong friendships. We made it to three Final Fours, but we never won the national championship – something I still regret after 20 years.

I thought about specialising in sports medicine as a way to combine my two passions, so I skipped around the globe, to the United States for an elective term in sports medicine at the University of Medicine and Dentistry in New Jersey, then back to Australia for my internship at Royal North Shore Hospital, where I rotated through different specialties. I quickly decided to follow a career in surgery, though I didn't yet know which speciality. Following my internship, I went to the UK for a residency in cardiothoracic surgery, plastic surgery, orthopedic surgery, and general surgery, and at Guy's Hospital in London, I asked a paediatric cardiac surgeon, Dr. David Anderson, whom I respected, what speciality he would choose if he had his time again. His immediate response was plastics.

When I asked why, he said "It's the only speciality where you get to work on the whole body, and it's the last general surgery left, since everything has become so specialised." I mulled this over while taking my surgical exams, and received my membership to the Royal College of Surgeons of England. That advice wasn't the only life-changing event during my tenure at Guy's: it was there I met Jodie, my future wife, who would later become the mother of our three wonderful girls, Rosie, Evie and Tessa, who are the inspiration for this book.

On returning to Sydney, I earned my board certification in *Plastic and Reconstructive Surgery* through the auspices of the Royal Australasian College of Surgeons (RACS), and then returned to London to complete a fellowship in microsurgical reconstruction for breast and head and neck cancer at Charing Cross Hospital and Imperial College. The next stop on my surgical training journey took me to Stockholm, Sweden, for a fellowship in cosmetic surgery with renowned plastic surgeon Dr. Per Heden and his team at Akademikliniken (AK), the largest private cosmetic surgery clinic in Europe.

I now divide my time between my private practice in Sydney, and the Prince of Wales Hospital, the Royal Hospital for Women and the Sydney Children's Hospital in Randwick, where I perform microsurgical reconstruction on cancer and trauma patients. I also sit on the National Education Board for training future plastic surgeons, and am currently the Chairperson for Training Plastic Surgery Residents in NSW.

My decision to become a plastic surgeon turned out to be the right one, because my job is helping people feel better about themselves. I hope that *Normal* will do the same for you or a loved one. I hope it sparks a conversation between parents and daughters who are suffering from body image issues. I want them to know that how they look is not their fault. Like the patients who share their stories in this book, I want to empower young women to reclaim their self-esteem, which may mean altering something they don't like about themselves. I want all girls to know that beauty is about confidence, not perfection. So before you or your child have any work done on the outside, make sure that the necessary work has been done from within. Plastic surgeons are a bit like architects – the best and most beautiful structures are built on strong foundations.

If you are a parent of a child who is depressed or being bullied, encourage them to share their thoughts about their appearance with you. Sometimes just naming a feeling can make a young person feel less alone. If they truly want to change something on their face or body, go with them for a professional evaluation. You wouldn't think twice about seeing an orthodontist to get braces to improve a smile. Similarly, plastic surgery can treat other physical issues that cause emotional distress.

## A BRIEF HISTORY OF PLASTIC AND RECONSTRUCTIVE SURGERY

There are many mysteries and misconceptions surrounding plastic surgery, and believe me, I've heard them all. So before I discuss the reasons so many girls and young women want to feel normal, here is some historical background. Contrary to popular belief, the 'plastic' in plastic surgery has nothing to do with implants; it comes from the Greek 'plastikos', meaning to mould or form. Plastic surgery can be used in nearly unlimited ways to achieve both reconstructive and aesthetic goals.

## ANCIENT ORIGINS

The practice dates back to ancient India, but evolved during the Roman Empire and Renaissance. In India c.600 BC, nose mutilation was used to punish and humiliate thieves, adulterers, and prisoners. The first to repair these injuries were the Koomas, a caste of Northern Indian priests, who were potters by trade. They used neighbouring tissues from the cheek and forehead to recreate the nose, and established principles that are the basis of modern-day rhinoplasty – aka nose jobs.

The foundation upon which all surgery is built is anatomy. If we don't know what defines normal, how can we create it when presented with the abnormal? Medical students dissect cadavers as part of their anatomy education. This was not always the case. During the early Roman Empire, Claudius Galen rose to prominence as a physician, anatomist, author, and philosopher. Because dissection was forbidden by Roman law, Galen gained insight into human anatomy while treating gladiators' combat wounds. His description of over 300 muscles and nerves helped generations of surgeons care for patients with congenital – or present at birth – and traumatic injuries.

Once the anatomy of a region is understood, the next step for surgeons is the safe manipulation of that anatomy to restore a normal appearance. Aulus Cornelus Celsus, one of the greatest Roman medical writers, detailed everything from repair of severed arteries to how surgery can address defects of the ears, lips, and nose in his book *De Medicina*. Many of the principles of modern-day plastic surgery, including the placement of incisions and wound management, were first established in Celsus's seminal work, and continue to be relevant today.

## UNIVERSITIES

The founding of the university as a centre of knowledge was key to educating physicians about surgical techniques. By the 12th century, cadaver dissection and the study of anatomy were central elements of medical education, using many of the same principles established over 1,000 years earlier by the Indians.

Gaspare Tagliacozzi (1545–1599) was a professor of surgery at Bologna University in Italy, and published extensively on nasal reconstruction.

He popularised the use of tissue from a distant body site in reconstructive surgery. The Tagliacozzi flap, or arm flap as it became known as, involved using the arm as a donor for the reconstruction of a recipient part of the body – in this case the nose. Tagliacozzi was one of the first to systematise the practice of reconstructive surgery, earning him the title of founder of modern-day plastic surgery, but following his death in 1599, the Catholic Church shunned these methods of reconstructive surgery as interfering with the work of God. Unfortunately, this Church decree set many of Tagliacozzi's innovative medical advances back 300 years.

## THE GOLDEN AGE OF PLASTIC SURGERY

The 19th century was the golden age of plastic surgery. There was a resurgence of nasal reconstruction, for example, with Carl Ferdinand von Gräfe's *Rhinoplasty: or the Art of Reconstructing the Nose*. Its publication established nasal reconstruction and rhinoplasty as central tenets in plastic surgery, and is still appreciated today. Then two major medical advances, skin grafting (1804) and anaesthesia (1846), revolutionised surgical procedures. Skin grafting has become one of the most widely used procedures to repair wounds in nearly every dimension of plastic surgery.

Similarly, advances in breast reconstruction were made in 1893 by Austrian-German surgeon Vincenz Czerny, who performed the first reconstructive breast augmentation on a patient with a benign breast mass. After the mass was removed, there was a significant size disparity between the two breasts, which Czerny corrected by removing a benign fat-based tumour from the patient's back, and using it to reconstruct her breast. This is the first documented reconstructive breast augmentation.

## WORLD WARS AND THE GUINEA PIG CLUB

Modern-day techniques were developed in the 20th century to treat injuries from World Wars I and II. The trench warfare of World War I resulted in a surge of soldiers returning home with devastating facial wounds, which prompted a collaboration between general surgery, otolaryngology, and oral surgery to address the bones, muscles, and skin that give the facial skeleton its structure. Sir Harold Gillies, an otolaryngologist from New Zealand who cared for many soldiers in France, established a centre for the management of facial traumatic injuries at Queen's Hospital, Sidcup, in South East London, on his return to the United Kingdom.

Later, during World War II, New Zealand-born Archibald McIndoe, a plastic surgeon and cousin of Sir Harold, moved to the Queen Victoria Hospital in East Grinstead, Sussex, to care for victims of wartime injuries. There he met Tom Gleave, a British fighter pilot who had sustained head-to-toe burns after his plane was shot down. McIndoe committed himself to providing comprehensive reconstructive care to Gleave, and pioneered methods of post-burn reconstruction. Gleave and other patients suffering from burn wounds were treated in Ward Three of the Queen Victoria Hospital, and he set up a drinking club so injured soldiers would find comfort in their shared experiences. Since they were many of the first patients to undergo such innovative procedures, they called themselves the Guinea Pig Club, led by Gleave, the chief guinea pig. In the years that followed, the Guinea Pig Club expanded its activities to rehabilitation and supporting patients in their re-entry and re-assimilation into society. Their influence was such that the local population of East Grinstead grew to embrace these men, and became known as "the town that never stared."

## THE EXPANSION OF COSMETIC SURGERY

Throughout the 20th century, the increase in training programs, scientific societies, and academic journals aided in the rapid expansion of plastic and reconstructive surgery as a speciality. Across the world, plastic surgeons became a central part of the hospital system treating patients with physical trauma or congenital anomalies, and eventually the speciality evolved to help patients who sought aesthetic treatments, such as noses, ears, eyes, excess weight, sagging chins, breast increases/reductions, and other procedures that I discuss in this book.

Whatever your issue may be, whether you are born with a physical abnormality or there is something you dislike about your appearance, for most people it's not about looking flawlessly beautiful – it's about fitting in. Humans are social animals, and we want to fit in so we can run with the pack. It's devastating to be teased or ostracised for something we have no control over, which is why I consider it a privilege to help people feel normal – which makes them feel better about themselves and, by extension, their lives.

If you are a parent, it never hurts to remind your daughters that they are far more than their looks. The self-criticism that comes from their reflection in the mirror or what they see in social media can be mitigated by a simple "I love you exactly as you are." And if you make a joint decision to change something about their appearance that they just can't live with, let them know that you will continue to love their new normal.

Here's the letter I wrote to my own daughters that eventually led to my writing this book.

> *Dear Girls,*
>
> *I love being your father. After the three of you were born, people would ask me if we would try again for a boy. I always told them "If we have a fourth, I would want another girl." I love that you are affectionate, caring, determined, and kind. I wanted to write this book before you reached puberty to let you know that beauty and power are about confidence. They're about being comfortable in your own skin. "Confidence is beautiful" was the mantra I chose for my practice when it first opened years ago. I like to think that I help people feel more confident for a living. Here are some things I want you to remember on your journey to adulthood.*

*My job as a father is to make you self-sufficient members of society. I will know I've been successful if I am rendered obsolete in this role. My goal is to establish a code of conduct to help you become independent women.*

*No one is perfect and there are things you can't control. You can't control who your parents are, where you are from, your race, your height or your skin colour. Don't focus on things you can't control. I never want you to be ashamed of your body or any part of it. But if you are insecure about a particular physical trait, there is a ladder of small steps you can take. Start with the lowest rung and work your way up the ladder if you feel you still need to. This could be as simple as owning your decision to accept yourself as you are. Or maybe the first step is a diet, exercise and lifestyle changes. Surgery should always be the last option for change, but sometimes it is the only option, as in developmental conditions.*

*Like you, your mum was one of three sisters, and she tells me I don't understand how difficult it is to be a teenage girl. I agree. The challenges and stresses for teenage girls are far greater than those of boys. For one, your bodies change monthly and cyclically. I have countless patients who tell me that their breast size fluctuates throughout their cycle, sometimes up to half a bra cup. Another factor conspiring against teenage girls is that many of your role models have had surgical enhancements – believe me, I know when this is the case – and their status is based on physical appearance. Male role models, on the other hand, are often athletes who are judged more on their sporting prowess than their looks. This is a generalisation, of course, and role modelling is changing with greater coverage of female athletes and businesswomen. So choose your role models wisely.*

*I want your journey to adulthood to be a smooth one, but I know that you will have challenges in life. Overcoming one obstacle, be it physical or emotional, doesn't mean you won't have others. It's like climbing a mountain. Scaling one peak simply means you are worthy of climbing another and then another. Succeeding at climbing one mountain doesn't take you to a mystical valley of no challenges, but rather towards other summits to conquer. Everyone fails multiple times, but you are only a loser if you blame others and accept none of the responsibility. Being a winner is not about getting a prize or a medal; it's about evolving, learning, not giving up, and having a purpose in life. Remember, it's hard to beat someone who never gives up.*

*Whatever problem you are having, whether it's body image, personal, or academic, and no matter how difficult it seems at the time, it is not a unique misfortune selected especially for you. There are no conspiracies out to get you and no one cares for your excuses. Never blame your problems on being a girl, not being smart enough, or looking a certain way. Adopt a growth mindset that you are not limited by your gender, ethnicity or physical status.*

*I asked your grandmother Zozo what her goals were for me and my brother growing up. She said what all parents really want for their children is that they are happy. This couldn't be more true, because with happiness comes confidence. And confidence is beautiful!*

*With love,*

*Dad*

Note: Names with asterisks have been changed to protect privacy.

CHAPTER ONE

# WHAT'S NORMAL ANYWAY?

Unless you're perfect – and no one is – it's absolutely normal to have a few physical traits that don't please you. Teens have grown up in a world where counting the number of likes on Instagram, watching porn, and obsessing about how they look as opposed to who they are as a person is normal. And parents worry about what they should do to help their daughters become healthy, informed adults.

This chapter aims to spark a conversation about what's normal, starting with some facts that may challenge preconceived notions about gender. I also explain what's normal – and what's not – during the developmental stages of puberty and adolescence. The biological changes that occur at this time are often accompanied by emotional and social changes, some of which I address as well. I trust young people to come to their own thoughtful conclusions if given the right information. One thing is certain however: what you see on TikTok, YouTube, TV, in the movies, or in fashion magazines is not the standard to which you should compare yourself – or anyone else for that matter. I write more about the impact of social and other media on self-confidence in *Your selfie image*, Chapter Eight on page 143.) For now, read on for some things to consider when asking what's normal anyway?

## THE NEW GENDER NORMS

Nowadays, lots of people (and nearly 3% of teens, according to a recent university study) identify as something other than the way they were born, with nonbinary and many other labels fast becoming the norm. Gender, like sexuality, is a spectrum, and many people fall within one end of it or the other. Today it is about how a person feels and how they choose to identify. The different gender identities include transgender, gender neutral, nonbinary, agender, pangender, genderqueer, a combination of these, and more. It can be confusing, so if you're not sure how someone wishes to identify, it's okay to ask what pronouns they prefer to avoid misgendering.

Whilst the sex assigned to you at birth is based on your genitalia, your gender can be about your lived experience, so when we talk about gender identity, we're talking about a person's deeply felt understanding of who they are. The following is a guide to the most commonly used terms for the new gender norms:

### *Gender expression*

This is the way a person expresses their gender through dress, hairstyle, or behaviour. Some present their gender in a way that fits societal expectations of male or female identity (i.e. female = high heels and dresses, male = suits and ties); others express in nontraditional ways. If someone feels uncomfortable revealing their gender identity in public, their outward appearance and behaviour may not reflect how they identify.

### *Sexual orientation*

You've probably seen or heard of LGBTQ+, which stands for Lesbian, Gay, Bisexual, Trans, Queer, and more, but because sexual orientation often gets mixed up in gender identity, it's worth talking about here. Sexual orientation, meaning the gender we're attracted to, is separate from our own gender identity. As YouTuber Brendan Jordan explained "Sexuality is who you go to bed with, and gender identity is who you go to bed as."

People sometimes make assumptions about a person's sexual orientation based on their gender identity – like assuming that transgender people are automatically gay. In truth, you can be a transgender woman who is attracted to other women and identifies as a lesbian, or you can be attracted to men and identify as straight. When it comes to sexual orientation and gender, a good rule of thumb is to avoid assumptions.

### *Nonbinary*

Until recently, an online search for nonbinary would have yielded few to no results. Fortunately, society has become far more accepting of fluidity,

## BRIDGETTE LUNDY-PAINE

Whilst shooting the third season of the Netflix series *Atypical*, Brigette Lundy-Paine, who played the spirited high school track star Casey, came out as nonbinary. "I had these experiences playing Casey that have been huge in discovering my gender," the actor told Us Weekly. "Since coming out, I've felt fear and relief when entering new spaces – fear that I'll make those around me uncomfortable, but relief that I no longer have to explain that I just don't *like* makeup and that this *particular* dress is just a little too tight."

not just in sexuality, but in gender identity too. Nonbinary is an umbrella term for people who identity as neither male nor female, and you can be nonbinary and also identify with other labels on this list. People will use she/her or he/him pronouns depending on which end of the gender spectrum they identify as, or gender-neutral pronouns like they/them or ze/hir (pronounced *zee* and *here*). You can use these pronouns in the same way you'd use a gendered pronoun like he or him in a sentence. It can take some getting used to at first, but using the right pronouns goes a long way toward making people feel comfortable. Questions about pronoun preference are now showing up on forms and applications (Australia issues nonbinary passports), and many teachers and professors ask their students what pronouns they use on the first day of school.

### *Queer*

Queer is a catch-all term used by some in the LGBTQ+ community when discussing gender identities and sexual preference. Queer can mean different things to different people, and many LGBTQ+ folks have appropriated the word to self-identify as a way to combat its use as a slur. If you are heterosexual, however, it's best to avoid using the term.

### *Cisgender*

Cisgender or cis describes people whose gender identity corresponds with their birth sex. So if you are biologically a girl and identify as female, or biologically a man and identify as male, you are cisgender.

### *Cishet*

Cishet is the term for people who are both cisgender and heterosexual.

### *Transgender/trans*

Transgender people do not identify with the sex they were assigned at birth. A transgender or trans person may have transitioned to their personal gender identity, be in the process of transitioning, or not be transitioning at all. Sex reassignment surgery can be done for those who want to transition from female to male or male to female. The procedures include hormone treatments, and are usually performed by a team of specialists, including gynecologists, urologists, pelvic pain specialists, and reconstructive plastic surgeons like me.

Though some transgender people also identify as nonbinary and use they/them pronouns, most identify as either male or female. Be sure to use the person's correct pronouns to avoid misgendering them. Again, it's okay to ask about pronouns if you're unsure. Tens of thousands of gender affirming surgeries are performed each year with great success. One of my transgender patients, Armani, shares her experience below. People like Armani are happier when they can be their authentic selves, and don't feel trapped in another body.

## Armani, 19, Byron Bay

*"I just want to be normal; it's the most important thing to me."*

"When I was six or seven I knew that I wasn't comfortable as a boy. I was pretty unhappy and stressed out as a child; I didn't quite understand what was wrong with me. I felt like I was trapped in the wrong body. I'd dress up as a girl around the house, but never in public. By the time I was 13, I knew I wanted to be a girl. I did a lot of research online and called a few surgeons to ask about the operations. I told a few of my high school friends that I wanted to transition. They weren't really surprised. When I told my parents they were shocked at first, as any parent would be, but they came around eventually. I'm an adopted only child, and they were supportive of my wishes because they wanted me to be happy.

Last year I went to my GP, who gave me a referral to a psychiatrist. That doctor referred me to an endocrinologist who prescribed hormones, which is the first step in the process. A few months after that, I saw Dr. Moradi for the breast implants, which I had done when I was 18. I love having breasts!

## LAVERNE COX

*"I just got to a point where I was sick of lying to myself."*

Actress Laverne Cox, best known for her role in *Orange is the New Black*, has been a trailblazer for the transgender community. Her frequent media appearances have led to a growing conversation about transgender culture, especially transgender women of colour. She is the first transgender person to be on the cover of *Time* magazine, and to be nominated for a Primetime Emmy. She is also the first trans woman to have a wax likeness in Madame Tussauds. Cox told a reporter that if it weren't for Tina Sparkles and all of the transgender women she met in the nightclub scene of New York City, she might not have ended up going to get her first hormone shot to start her medical transition. "I just got to a point where I was sick of lying to myself," she said. "I was sick of not being in the truth. I think we all get to a point in our lives where we can no longer lie to ourselves, so we have to stand in our truths and begin to manifest that truth outwardly… And if you're not there yet, you'll get there. It's a process, it's a search."

## RUBY ROSE

*"I am very gender fluid."*

Australian model and actress Ruby Rose has been open about her gender fluidity, and even released a short film about it back in 2014. You can see it on YouTube. "I am very gender fluid and feel more like I wake up every day sort of gender neutral," she told News Corp Australia. Rose said she was frequently bullied and beaten up by classmates at school. One incident was so bad, she had to be hospitalised and could not return to school for five days. "I got beaten up by about four girls and one guy in front of about 50 people," she recalls."They hit me on the head with metal chairs at a café, and they threw things at me. They punched me. I ended up with lacerations, big bruises, and concussion."

In 2003, Rose came in second in a modelling competition for an Australian teen magazine. Being in the spotlight brought out her rebellious streak. If people criticised her tattoos, she'd get more. If they commented on her shaved head, she'd dye it pink. "I wasn't anti-modelling," she says, "I was anti being told that I had to look a certain way, and that how I looked wasn't good enough. If anything it just made me kind of bolder and stronger."

I'm an R&B singer and a high-fashion editorial model, and now I can wear so many things that I wasn't able to wear before my boob job. I feel so much more confident. I always looked feminine, but now there's no question that when people look at me, they're looking at a woman.

I'm planning to go to Melbourne in six months to have the sex affirming operation. That operation is a much bigger deal. I'm excited about getting it all done, and I want to do it as quickly as possible. Now that I've started changing my life, things have gotten so much better.

I'd tell anyone who is considering a transition to do it as quickly as possible so they can feel better about themselves. I'm fiercely independent, so I'm okay on my own, but I encourage people to get the support of others who've been through it if they need it. I look forward to wearing bikinis, going to the beach, and not having to worry about excess baggage. I just want to be normal; it's the most important thing to me. I think that's what transitioning is all about – being able to fit in and not standing out anymore. The last thing trans people want to do is to stand out."

### *Gender fluid*

Someone who identifies as gender fluid may fluctuate between genders or express multiple genders at the same time. Their gender can vary depending on the day or circumstance.

### *Gender neutral/agender*

Someone who feels they are neither male nor female may identify as gender neutral or agender. People who identify as gender neutral or agender may prefer to dress androgynously, but you don't have to be androgynous to be agender or vice versa.

### *Intersex*

Intersex is a general term used to describe someone who is born with genitalia that has some male characteristics and some female characteristics. This includes what can't be seen on the outside, such as a

## ANGEL HAZE

Angel Haze garnered fame and fans with her breakout rap album *Dirty Gold*. She identifies as agender, and revealed in 2016 that she doesn't have a preference for pronouns. "If you call me him or her it doesn't matter to me," she told a reporter from *The Evening Standard*. "I don't consider myself of any sex. I consider myself an experience."

uterus. Surgeries may be performed on infants to make their body fit the binary definition of male or female, but are frequently delayed until the patient is old enough to choose a gender.

*Two Spirit*

Two Spirit comes from Indigenous peoples in Canada/Turtle Island/North America. It can mean a person who walks between genders, one who carries the gifts of both males and females, or one who is gender neutral.

**What parents can do**

Many parents may be unsure of how to support their teens who are confused about their gender identity. A Stanford University research team asked 25 teens and their parents for their thoughts on this, and the teens said they appreciate having parents who use their preferred name and pronoun, as well as knowing that their parents are emotionally available and listen to their concerns. Interestingly, the teens rated their parents as being more supportive than the parents rated themselves. The findings, which were published in the *Journal of Adolescent Health*, show the importance of the parent-child relationship, and the willingness of parents to understand their teen.

## WHAT'S NORMAL DURING PUBERTY?

Puberty is a time of physical development and changes: your feet and hands get bigger, more baby teeth fall out, your face may be spotted with acne, and you mature sexually. These physical changes are triggered by hormones, chemical agents that travel around the body and send messages to cells to perform specific actions. In boys, there is an increased production of testosterone, a male sex hormone, whilst girls have an increased production of the female hormone estrogen. These hormones can cause emotional fluctuations, such as mood swings that make you feel exuberant one moment and sullen the next.

It's also normal to have a growth spurt during this time that causes the body to crave additional energy from food. It's not unusual for a teen to have a voracious appetite during puberty, which is why parents jokingly complain that their kids are eating them out of house and home. Increased appetites tend to be more common in boys because of the surge in testosterone, and in most cases an active teenager will burn the extra calories, but teens don't always make the healthiest food choices. If you start gaining too much weight from sweets, salty snacks or junk food, you may want to switch to a healthier diet or talk to a doctor or nutritionist.

## WHAT HAPPENS TO GIRLS DURING PUBERTY?

Puberty frequently starts earlier for girls than boys. Here's a typical timeline:

- Puberty begins between 8 and 13 years old
- First puberty change is breast development (see *Breast wishes*, Chapter Three on page 53)
- Pubic hair appears shortly after breast development. The first growth produces soft hair in a small area around the genitals. This eventually becomes darker and coarser, and over time it may spread to the thighs and, in some cases, as far up as the stomach
- Armpit hair appears at about the age of 12
- Menstrual periods begin between 10 and 16½ years old. (More on this in *Parts down under*, Chapter Five on page 91.)

## DELAYED PUBERTY

When a teen goes through body changes later than usual, it's called delayed puberty. For girls, it means no breast development by the age of 13, or no menstrual periods by the age of 16.

### *What causes delayed puberty?*

Don't be concerned if you are a late bloomer who happens to start puberty after most girls your age. Being a late bloomer is the most common reason for delayed puberty. It's not caused by a medical problem and it usually doesn't require treatment. Try to be patient, because late bloomers usually start puberty on their own and catch up with their friends. That said, there are several medical causes for delayed puberty, including a condition called Kallmann syndrome. People with this condition are unable to smell, and have low luteinizing (LH) and follicle-stimulating hormones (FSH). Low levels of both LH and FSH may indicate secondary ovarian failure, which means another part of your body may have caused ovarian failure, and be the result of problems in the areas of your brain that produce hormones, such as the pituitary gland.

In some cases, girls don't start having periods because their uterus has not developed properly, or they may have too much of a hormone called prolactin, a condition called polycystic ovary syndrome (PCOS). Another medical condition that only affects females is called Turner syndrome, where one of the X (sex) chromosomes is missing or partially missing. Turner syndrome can produce a slew of medical and developmental problems, including stunted growth, failure of the ovaries to develop, and heart defects. It may be diagnosed before birth, during infancy, or in early childhood, and in girls with mild symptoms the diagnosis is delayed until the teen or young adult years. Those diagnosed with Turner syndrome will need ongoing medical care by a variety of specialists, such as a pediatric endocrinologist. If you are concerned about delayed puberty, or started to develop and suddenly stopped, consult a doctor.

### *How does a doctor check for delayed puberty?*

A physician can check for abnormal development by doing blood tests for hormone levels. The doctor will measure your height and weight, and take an X-ray of your hand to see if the bones are developing more slowly than usual. Sometimes doctors can see signs of puberty that you may not have

# OTHER CAUSES OF DELAYED PUBERTY

The following are some less common causes of delayed puberty:

- Medical conditions that keep the intestines from absorbing nutrients from food, such as celiac disease or inflammatory bowel disease
- Malnutrition due to an eating disorder such as anorexia
- Problems with the pituitary or thyroid glands, which make hormones that help children grow and develop
- Some cancer treatments that affect sex hormone production
- Medicines that decrease appetite, such as stimulants for attention deficit hyperactivity disorder (ADHD).

noticed, and in some cases a brain scan such as an MRI will show problems with the pituitary gland. Girls may need a sonogram to see if their uterus and ovaries are developing as they should.

***What's the treatment for delayed puberty?***

Sometimes doctors will prescribe short-term hormone therapy to help teens start developing. Girls may be prescribed estrogen pills or skin patches, and some teens need long-term hormone therapy if they are not able to make normal amounts of estrogen.

## THE TEEN BRAIN

During adolescence, enormous changes take place in the brain, which is not fully developed until about the age of 25 although it has stopped growing in size. This explains why a teenager's judgement and decision-making skills are not always the best. In fact, recent research has found that a teen brain actually works differently from an adult's. Adults think with the prefrontal cortex, the front part of the brain responsible for rational thought, which is one of the last regions to mature. Here are some other facts about the teen brain:

- *The brain reaches full size in early adolescence.* A girl's brain reaches its maximum size when she is about 11 years old. A boy's brain is fully grown when he is about 14. Size does not matter when it comes to intelligence
- *The teen brain is ready to learn and adapt.* The teen brain has lots of plasticity, which means it can easily change, adapt, and respond to its environment. Certain activities, such as exercise, art, and learning to speak another language or how to play an instrument, help the brain mature and strengthen.
- *Teens need more sleep.* Research shows that melatonin levels in the blood are naturally higher later at night and drop later in the morning in teens than in most children and adults. This difference could explain why many teens stay up late and struggle with getting up in the morning.

If you find it difficult to wake up in the morning without an alarm, you're probably not getting enough rest. Try going to bed earlier, and unplugging from your phone and other devices one hour before lights out. Sleep deprivation can impair your memory, decision-making, focus, and creativity – all of which are necessary for success at school. Playing catch up on the weekends by getting extra sleep will only make it harder to regulate during the week. If you are feeling draggy and foggy brained during the day, you are probably sleep deprived.

- *Some mental disorders may emerge during adolescence.* Ongoing changes in the brain, along with physical, emotional, and social changes, can make teens vulnerable to mental health problems. The big changes going on in the brain is the reason mental disorders such as schizophrenia, bipolar disorder, and eating disorders emerge at this time.
- *Teen brains are vulnerable to stress.* Because the brain is still developing, teens may respond to stress differently to adults, which may lead to stress-related mental disorders such as anxiety and depression. Although mood swings are normal, depression can interfere with the ability to function. It affects 20% of teens by the time they're adults, according to the Physicians' Review Network. Signs of depression include: a lack of interest in activities and subjects you've once enjoyed, withdrawal, a significant change in weight or appetite, fatigue and low energy, feelings of worthlessness and guilt, cutting or pulling out hair, a drop in grades, irritability, and suicidal thoughts. If you are depressed, don't try to go it alone – tell someone: a friend, parent, or a trusted adult. A combination of talk therapy and medication is the go-to treatment for teen depression.

## LET'S TALK ABOUT LUCY

Lucy Suffern, my best friend in high school, took her own life tragically on the 21st April, 1997, at the age of 19. She had suffered from depression all of her brief life. I vividly remember the evening I heard about her death: I was in second-year medical school and I got home to find my friend Briony at the door. She had also been one of Lucy's classmates, and she sat me down and told me that Lucy had taken her own life in her dorm at university in Townsville, where she was studying marine biology.

I had first learned of Lucy's condition 18 months earlier when we were sitting for our HSC together. It was July 1995, and Lucy had gone down to Melbourne to visit her aunt. When I saw her again, I noticed she had bandages on her wrists, and I naïvely believed her when she claimed she had had an accident washing dishes. I even remember joking that I thought she had tried to harm herself. That was how absurd I thought it was that she would do such a thing. This pretense was short-lived as she eventually revealed the extent of her depression to me. Before that first suicide attempt, I had spent the best part of six years of high school with her, travelling to and from home to school without suspecting a thing. Lucy later confided in me during these dark days that her depression and anxiety had started when she was 12, and for most of her life she fought the battle by herself with no help.

Three months later, the night before the first HSC exam, I got a call from the school and her parents that Lucy had attempted suicide again, this time with a blowdryer in the bathtub. It was crystal clear Lucy was not fit to sit the exams, and she came over to our house and stayed the night. Torn between my studies and a friend, we talked all night long. The next day, driving to the English exam, my least favourite subject, I had a car accident. I ran up the back of another driver. Fortunately no one was hurt, and the driver was a solid human being. He saw the frantic state I was in, and he took my parents' home phone number – no mobile phones back then. He said if there was any damage he couldn't fix, he would call. I am still waiting for his call. I sat the exams and, by some divine intervention, scored well enough to get into medical school.

Lucy had sought professional help after her first suicide attempt, and I honestly thought she was cured by the time we went to our high school formal together six weeks later. We were both in relationships with other people, but it made sense to end high school as partners for the graduation ball. Reflecting on those days, I am not quite sure why I was so naïve as to think her depression and demons had been cured. Her diagnosis was, I thought, a fleeting one – something that could be cured with a pill and a hug. Maybe a part of me wanted to believe it was attention-seeking behaviour, because I had no reference to compare it to. Depression and suicide were not talked about at all in the mid-nineties, and there was no support structure for patients, friends, and family like there is today.

The following year, I started medical school and Lucy took a year off from her studies. Whilst we didn't see as much of each other, we remained close. Well, as close as you can be when going down different paths. I recall interviewing Lucy for social studies and psychology assignments on her battles with mental health. To me, all seemed well. In 1997, Lucy was enrolled at James Cook University in Townsville, which is three hours by plane from Sydney on the northern point of Australia. We stayed in contact, and the first email I ever sent was to Lucy from the Mechanical Engineering building at UNSW, which had the only computers in the university where you could access your email account. I believe it all began to unravel again when she left Sydney and the safety of her friends and family to pursue her childhood dream of being a marine biologist. Alone and isolated on that fateful day, Lucy finally succeeded in ending her suffering.

Anyone who has ever lost a friend or loved one through suicide has probably experienced a multitude of feelings, none of which help bring them back. To be honest, these emotions didn't help me make sense of my loss. I felt sadness at the passing of a gentle and pure soul whom I will never share moments and stories with again. I felt the sense of a life wasted – one that would never live up to my expectations. I felt shocked that things were so bad for her that the only escape was to take her own life.

I read a great quote on Instagram about the despair that those suffering from depression feel. The post shows harrowing images of people jumping

# EMMA, 18

*"I'm not suicidal, but I don't want this existence anymore."*

"I'm not really functioning outside of working/shopping for my family right now. I can't tell if I'm mildly depressed or just reacting normally to what's going on in the present and everything that has happened in my past to make me the messed up and stunted person that I am today. Either way, I'm struggling to get much of anything done, even things I enjoy, and I cry an awful lot. I'm not suicidal, but I don't want this existence anymore.

My social anxiety has also gone up a gear thanks to my low mood and incredibly low self-esteem. Speaking of which, working at the supermarket really hasn't been great for my self-esteem. I get yelled at and treated like an idiot by one of the managers just for asking basic questions. I know it's almost definitely her rather than me, given that absolutely everyone in my department constantly mentions how horrible she is with other people. However, when you combine this with having to deal with a handful of rude customers, and then add in the fact that I seem incapable of having even a basic conversation with my co-workers, and don't feel like I fit in with them at all or that anyone there likes me, I'm sure you can see how this would grind down any belief in myself. I have some serious concerns about my ability to function due to my non-existent self-confidence."

to their death from the burning inferno of the Twin Towers after the 9/11 terrorist attacks in New York. It said that people suffering from depression who commit suicide are standing on the edge of an abyss. They have two grim choices: to be burnt alive or jump. For those of us who are lucky not to have these ideations, it is hard to fathom someone taking their own life, but to those who suffer from depression, when seen in the context of the Twin Towers, jumping from a great height is the better of the two evils. This concept helped me understand Lucy's mindset, and that the torture she must have been going through was far worse than the reality of taking her own life.

Once all of the stages of grief, sadness, and shock had subsided, the overriding feeling that has stayed with me for the last 25 years is guilt. Guilt that I didn't do more, guilt that, as her best friend, I wasn't there for her, guilt that my life has moved on, guilt that as time passes her memory and our moments together have faded. Even now, after all these years, I have the same feeling. Whilst not as raw and real as it was when I was a teenager, it still exists and nags away at my soul.

My advice to my daughters, and to anyone reading this book who may have felt suicidal, is this: talk to someone. Whether it is you or a loved one who is suffering, talk freely, talk often, and talk forever. In the days, weeks, months, and even years after Lucy's passing, I never talked to anyone about my feelings. I internalised my emotions. All I wanted to do was talk – not to someone about my grief, not necessarily to have them listen or help – just as a sounding board for my thoughts.

Mental illness is not an acute ailment like a twisted ankle that heals itself. It is a chronic condition that needs nurturing and support. Looking back, my mistakes with Lucy are glaring. I assumed, because she stopped talking about her sadness, the disease had been cured. I now know better. Don't keep your feelings bottled up inside you. Tell someone, and get treatment so you can get better.

## What parents can do

Here are somes tips for communicating with a depressed teen, which I realise can be difficult, especially if they are withdrawing from you and others:

- **Focus on listening, not lecturing.** When talking with your teen, resist the urge to criticise or pass judgement once they begin to talk. The important thing is that your child is communicating. Simply letting your teen know that you're there for them, fully and unconditionally, is a great step forward. Set aside time each day to talk – time when you're not distracted or trying to multitask. Driving in the car is also a great place to talk as both of you are looking forward, and for some reason this is easier for teens – and, to be honest, adults too. Connecting face to face can play a big role in reducing your teen's depression. Remember, talking about depression or your teen's feelings will not make the situation worse.
- **Be gentle, but persistent.** Don't give up if they shut you out at first. Talking about depression can be very tough for teens, just as it is for adults. They may have a hard time expressing what they're feeling, even if they want to. Respect your child's comfort level while emphasising that you are concerned and willing to listen.
- **Acknowledge their feelings.** Don't try to talk your teen out of depression, even if their feelings or concerns appear silly or irrational to you. Saying things like "it's not that bad" will come across as dismissive. Simply acknowledging your child's pain and sadness goes a long way in making them feel understood and supported.
- **Trust your gut.** If your teen claims nothing is wrong, but has no explanation for what is causing the depressed behaviour, trust your instincts. If your teen won't open up to you, consider asking a school counsellor, favourite teacher, coach, or a mental health professional. The goal is to get them talking, and it doesn't necessarily have to be to you. In fact it probably won't be you.

- **Encourage social connection.** Depressed teens often withdraw from their friends and the activities they used to enjoy. This isolation only makes depression worse, so do what you can to help your teen reconnect. Encourage them to go out with friends or invite friends over. Participate in activities that involve other families.
- **Try to reduce their social media use.** I write about this at length in the *Your Selfie Image*, Chapter Eight on page 143. Studies show that social media can make depression worse in teens. Encourage them to turn off their phone – or at least disable notifications – when socialising with friends, doing homework, and before going to bed. Set limits on screen time. You can set an example by not scrolling and texting at mealtimes or family gatherings.
- **Get your teen involved.** Suggest activities such as sports, after-school clubs, art, dance, music class, or volunteering for a cause they believe in. The best activities involve your teen's interests and talents, not yours. While your teen may be completely unmotivated at first, once they get involved in outside interests they will start to feel better.
- **Make physical health a priority.** Physical and mental health are inextricably connected. Depression is exacerbated by inactivity, lack of sleep, and poor nutrition. Unfortunately, teens are known for their unhealthy habits: staying up late, eating junk food, and spending hours on their phones and devices. As a parent, you can combat these behaviours by serving healthy meals, and establishing a supportive home environment.
- **Seek professional help, if needed.** Support and healthy lifestyle changes can make a world of difference for depressed teens, but it's not always enough. When depression is severe, don't hesitate to seek help from a mental health professional who is trained to work with teens. If necessary, medication may be a part of the treatment plan.

**Resource for depression support and suicide prevention**

- Call the SANE Help Centre at 1800 18 7263 or Lifeline Australia at 13 11 14.

CHAPTER TWO

# BODY DYSMORPHIA

As I said in the Introduction, one of the biggest fears I have for my daughters is that they will grow to hate something about their face or body. It is my fervent wish that my girls – and the readers of this book – be comfortable in their own skin. Sadly, this is not the case for those suffering from body dysmorphic disorder (BDD), which is a psychological condition that typically begins by the age of 12 or 13, continues through adolescence and, for some, into adulthood. One out of every 50 people suffers from body dysmorphia, according to the Cleveland Clinic. Other studies estimate between 2% of high schoolers, and 13–28% of college students have BDD.

People with BDD are obessessed with their appearance, overly critical of real or perceived flaws, and have severe distress that interferes with their personal, social, and professional lives. This preoccupation with their perceived appearance flaws frequently leads to depression, with as many as 80% of BDD sufferers having suicidal thoughts. Many seek cosmetic procedures, including 230,000 teens in 2017, according to the American Academy of Facial Plastic Surgery, some as young as 13. And more than half of all plastic surgery patients have BDD. If left untreated, body dysmorphia will grow stronger over time.

Body dysmorphia is especially prevalent amongst teens, who are convinced that something about their body or face is so ugly that it's the only thing their peers can see. In one of the largest studies of patients with BDD, the average age of onset was 16, although unhappiness with appearance began about 13. Although most people show signs of BDD in late adolescence, the majority of those do not get psychologically evaluated until their thirties.

Some parents may not recognise the difference between BDD and general teenage malaise. It is far more than the occasional "I hate my thighs" complaint though. Whilst it's not unusual for teens to dislike something about their appearance, those with BDD have an unwavering anxiety about one or more body parts. They spend hours in front of a mirror, exercise excessively, or get cosmetic procedures but are never satisfied with the results. The more convinced they are, the more distress and disruption they experience.

It may be surprising to learn that BDD affects men and women equally. Men who are preoccupied with their build and think their bodies are too small, too scrawny, or not pumped up enough have what's known as muscle dysmorphia. In most cases, men with muscle dysmorphia, also known as bigorexia or megarexia, already have large or muscular physiques and have an unrealistic view of their bodies. For three years, Veya Seekis, a psychology professor at Griffith University in Queensland, Australia, has been collecting data on the social media habits of 303 male undergraduates and 198 high school boys in Australia. She has found that exposure to images of archetypal masculine physiques was linked to low body esteem in young men, and an increased desire to become more muscular. "The more men view their bodies as objects for public display, the more they fear being negatively evaluated," Dr. Seekis told a reporter from *The New York Times*, "which so often triggers compulsive exercising and other 'healthy' behaviours that can end up having an impact on their well-being."

As a plastic surgeon who makes a living altering parts of the body and face that patients are unhappy with, it can be difficult to differentiate between someone with BDD and a so-called normal patient who simply wants to look and feel better. The Australian Medical Board has identified BDD as such a big issue that from the 1st of July 2023 it has made it compulsory for all patients seeking cosmetic surgery to have a BDD screen prior to their consultation. I see at least one patient a week who tells me they haven't been naked with the lights on in front of their partner for years. Some of these patients may have body dysmorphia, while others may simply have a negative body image.

One thing that's true of all patients with BDD, however, is that they are rarely, if ever, satisfied with the results after surgery. Patients who seek rhinoplasty – nose jobs – have the highest rate of BDD, as well as dissatisfaction with their procedures. In a 2013 Greek study, researchers assessed 166 rhinoplasty patients for BDD. The higher they scored on the BDD scale, the more disappointed they were with their results after surgery, and the lower their quality of life. Likewise, in a 2016 study from Brazil, between 40–57% of patients having rhinoplasty, abdominoplasty (aka tummy tucks), or facelifts had the highest rate of BDD.

Screening for body dysmorphia is one reason all Australians between the ages of 16 and 18 who plan to have cosmetic procedures must get a psychological assessment along with a mandatory three-month waiting period prior to surgery. The most common procedures teens have done are rhinoplasty, breast reduction, and tuberous breast reconstruction.

## SYMPTOMS OF BDD

- A preoccupation with a perceived flaw in appearance that is not noticed by or appears minor to others
- An overwhelming belief that a physical defect makes you ugly or deformed
- A belief that other people are mocking something about your appearance
- An inability to control behaviours aimed at fixing or hiding a perceived flaw, such as frequently checking in the mirror, grooming, or skin picking
- Hiding perceived flaws with hair styling, makeup, or clothes
- Constantly comparing your appearance with others
- Frequently seeking reassurance about your appearance from others
- Perfectionist tendencies
- Having cosmetic procedures that do not change your opinion of yourself
- Avoiding social situations.

Thinking excessively about perceived flaws can make it difficult to function, and also cause problems at school, work, and home. The most common features BDD sufferers fixate on include:

- Face, such as nose, complexion, wrinkles, acne, and other blemishes
- Hair, such as appearance, thinning, and baldness
- Skin and vein appearance
- Breast size
- Muscle size and tone
- Genitalia.

If you think you may have BDD, take this online questionnaire created by the Body Dysmorphic Foundation at https://bddfoundation.org/helping-you/questionnaires-do-i-have-bdd/. While only a trained health professional can make a diagnosis, the results can be used to measure the severity of symptoms before and after getting treatment, and give you feedback on whether or not your symptoms have improved with treatment.

## THREE DIAGNOSTIC CRITERIA FOR BODY DYSMORPHIC DISORDER

1. A preoccupation with an imagined or slight defect in appearance – if a slight physical defect is present, the person's degree of concern is extreme
2. Marked distress or impairment in social, occupational, or other areas
3. The preoccupation is not attributable to the presence of another psychiatric disorder such as anorexia nervosa

Whilst 1. is common amongst all patients seeking cosmetic plastic surgery, the other criteria may stand out to surgeons when assessing their patient's suitability for surgery. That said, the secrecy and shame that often accompanies BDD only adds to the difficulty in diagnosing this condition. One reason the disorder can go unrecognised is that people are often embarrassed and reluctant to tell their doctors about their concerns.

## BILLIE EILISH OPENS UP ABOUT BDD

Billie Eilish, the 18-year-old pop star, has been open about her body image issues. In a cover story for *Rolling Stone*, she said they started after she joined a competitive dance company at the age of 12, and ultimately became full-blown BDD: "That was the peak of my body dysmorphia," she said. "I couldn't look in the mirror at all… I couldn't speak and just be normal. When I think about it or see pictures of me then, I was so not OK with who I was." Eilish credits therapy with helping her overcome this and other mental health struggles.

As hard as it can be to diagnose BDD in the patients who desire cosmetic surgery, it's a red flag when someone repeatedly seeks plastic surgery for the same real or perceived physical defects. Another telltale sign is when a patient has seen multiple surgeons and claims "they won't operate on me because they don't think they can help me" or "they don't understand what I want."

The fact that BDD is under-diagnosed was confirmed by a 2017 Dutch university study. The study, which appeared in *Plastic and Reconstructive Surgery*, asked plastic surgeons, dermatologists, and other cosmetic professionals about their experiences with BDD. About two-thirds of the 173 respondents said they had encountered one to five patients with BDD in their practice over the past few years. Most said they either sometimes or often addressed body image problems while consulting with patients – but only 7% routinely did so. About 70% said they would refuse to perform cosmetic procedures on a patient they suspected of having BDD, and just under half said they worked with psychologists or psychiatrists. Approximately 16% of those surveyed also reported verbal altercations with patients, and 6% had been threatened with legal action. The bottom line is that BDD is something that surgeons need to be aware of and learn more about how to address properly.

Before any plastic surgery is performed, there should be a patient evaluation that includes a complete history and a focused physical exam. If a doctor suspects BDD based on an assessment of the patient's attitude, behaviour, and symptoms, they should refer them to a mental health professional who is trained to diagnose BDD. I would estimate I refer 5–10% of my patients to a BDD specialist, the majority of those seeking a rhinoplasty. In Australia, the medical regulators have enforced a three-month cooling-off period along with a psychologist's assessment for all patients under the age of 18 who wish to have cosmetic surgery as another measure to help protect patients from unnecessary discretionary surgery.

## WHAT CAUSES BODY DYSMORPHIC DISORDER?

Although the exact cause of BDD is not known, one theory suggests it may have something to do with certain areas of the brain that process information about appearance. The fact that BDD often occurs in people with major depression and anxiety indicates there may be a biological basis for the disorder. The neurobiological, psychological, and sociocultural factors explained below are also thought to play a role in the development of body dysmorphia.

### *Neurobiological*

There is some evidence to suggest that body dysmorphic disorder has a genetic underpinning. A study of 1,000 patients with BDD found 20% had at least one first-degree family member with it. Other studies suggest that BDD is more common in families of those diagnosed with obsessive-compulsive disorder (OCD), indicating that there may be a common genetic link between the disorders.

### *Psychological factors*

The cause of body dysmorphia can be explained by at least two psychological theories: cognitive and behavioural. A cognitive-behavioural perspective suggests the disorder comes from an interaction of cognitive thinking, emotions, and behaviours. Cognitive factors that appear in BDD include unrealistic attitudes about body image, perfection, and symmetry, focused attention on a perceived defect, increased self-monitoring for the presence of appearance flaws, and a belief that one's appearance is far less attractive than the ideal. From a behavioural perspective, BDD is thought to arise from comparing one's appearance to peers or to those seen in the media.

### *Sociocultural factors*

Sociocultural causes of body dysmorphia are often discovered when taking patients' social histories. For example, people can develop BDD if they are raised in a family that is rejecting, neglectful, and critical, especially of physical appearance. This is particularly the case during adolescence, the typical age of onset for this disorder, if someone is teased about the way they look. Ridicule may cause a person to question their appearance, even if it's not flawed. The emphasis on physical perfection in the media is another potential cause of negative body image, low self-esteem, and body dysmorphic disorder (see *Your Selfie Image,* Chapter Eight on page 143).

## HOW IS BODY DYSMORPHIC DISORDER TREATED?

Treatment for BDD can include a combination of the following therapies:

- *Psychotherapy.* A psychologist or psychotherapist treating someone with BDD will focus on changing the patient's thinking (cognitive therapy) and behaviour (behavioural therapy). The goal is to correct the false belief about the defect and to minimise the compulsive behaviour.
- *Medication.* Certain antidepressant medications called selective serotonin reuptake inhibitors (SSRIs) are used in treating BDD, as are antipsychotic medicines such as aripiprazole (Abilify), olanzapine (Zyprexa), or pimozide (Orap) either alone or in combination with an SSRI. At this writing, there is no FDA-approved drug specifically for the treatment of BDD.
- *Group and/or family therapy.* Family support is an important part of treatment. Family members who understand BDD and learn to recognise its signs and symptoms can help.

## CAN BDD BE SUCCESSFULLY TREATED?

The outlook is promising. Those who get treatment, and people with a strong support group, tend to do better in the long run, but because BDD is essentially a body image problem, cosmetic procedures are not recommended, as they yield no improvement or even aggravate the condition in as many as 95% of patients diagnosed with BDD.

When I see patients who are anxious about changing their appearance, and their expectations are unreasonable (e.g. "I want my partner to find me attractive" or "A nose job will get me the job of my dreams"), I tell them to rethink surgery, because in most cases they will be disappointed with the results.

The following emotionally haunting stories will give you an idea of what it's like to live with BDD:

### *Zoe

*"The mirror was my best friend and my worst enemy."*

I was in primary school when I first started thinking that I was skinny and awkward-looking. Somebody teased me in the playground, and someone else insisted that I needed tidying up, but I was already an insecure little girl. Life at home was unstable. I wanted so much to feel loved and accepted. I spent my childhood years feeling depressed, and started to believe that the key to happiness lay in my looking a certain way.

I would fan out my hair on the pillow at night, hoping my mother would pop her head around the corner and think what a beautiful daughter she had. In fact, I felt anything but. I was angry inside. I wet the bed and had terrible nightmares. I suffered from panic attacks. I felt like a disappointment. I felt weird. As I got older, school became a struggle. I was stuck in a rut of negative thinking about myself. Despite positive attention from friends and an aptitude for some subjects, I became entrenched in the belief that I was not good enough. I was allowing myself to be ruled by an ideal of unattainable perfection.

I looked to the mirror to help me cope with my difficult feelings. If I could only make myself appear a certain way then I would be okay. Or so my thinking went. I wore thermals underneath my clothes to bulk me out; I hid behind layers of make-up. I wore my hair a particular way to disguise all that

I saw wrong with me. The mirror was my best friend and my worst enemy. I gazed in it secretly, because the monster was always gazing back, keeping me locked in a cycle of preening and face-pulling. I would become quietly hysterical at the sight of a photograph of myself.

I believed I was a monster. I had to conceal my true identity from the world at any cost. So at the age of 15, when life should have been exciting and full of a sense of character-building experiences, I dropped out of school and, for an entire year, became a recluse. I lost touch with the world and life grew cold and lonely. All my time was spent gazing into the mirror, wondering why I couldn't look and be normal like everyone else.

At 16 I finally met someone, moved to London, and started working. People would offer up compliments and even tell me that I should be modelling. Although I thrived on positive attention when I was with others, later, alone at home, my hellish reality would dawn on me again. I felt like a fraud. I'd spend hours naked, just looking at myself, poking and prodding bits, preening, exercising, worrying that every additive in the food I ate was conspiring to make my skin uglier. I'd check my reflection from every angle, under every kind of light, always ending up back with my self-loathing and tears. My life was not so much about living as surviving. I didn't feel worthy of happiness. So many times I ran away, only to find that I couldn't get away from myself. With each new home, new area, new job, I'd vow that things would be different. I'd be different. But nothing changed.

I remember the day I first heard about body dysmorphic disorder. Flicking through a magazine, I came across an article with the heading "I Feel Too Ugly to Live". It spoke directly to me. As I started to read I had a sense of revelation, because I saw myself in this horrendous illness. Suddenly I wasn't alone, I wasn't crazy. I know some people struggle to believe they have this disorder, but for me there was no mistaking it. I went to get a professional opinion at the Priory in North London, and walked away determined that I'd kick arse with this disorder.

I tried various medications, eventually some counselling – I even visited a spiritual healer and tried prayer. I read up on the illness; I went online to raise awareness and to find other sufferers. Yes, some days I struggle and cry and get frustrated, because I don't feel good enough or presentable. It's to be expected; you pick yourself up and brush yourself down. I have found ways to keep my BDD demons under control, and to get enjoyment out of things I never could before.

What I most want to say is this: there is light at the end of the tunnel. It's a slow process reprogramming your brain to think differently so you eventually feel differently, but it's worth it! And it can even be fun getting to discover who you really are from the inside too, to see yourself changing for the better by developing new ways of thinking and being. I try to appreciate that beauty lies in imperfections and uniqueness.

### *Sue

*"I thought about my ugly appearance every moment of the day."*

I experienced symptoms of BDD from a very early age. I was always sensitive and self-conscious, and felt that I was different from the other girls. My confidence increased slightly when I reached my mid-teens and I was able to camouflage my appearance with make-up and straighten my hair. With the arrival of a few boyfriends and my marriage at 18, I felt a little more "normal," but by this time the obsessive behaviours had set in.

At 21 my marriage broke down and I became severely depressed. At that point BDD took over my life. I was so repulsed and disgusted by my appearance that I thought no one would ever want me again. My parents took me to the GP, who treated me for depression and prescribed Valium. The BDD and depression became so unbearable that I took an overdose, and was then referred to a psychiatrist. The next seven years of my life were spent in and out of hospital, trying countless different medications.

But the symptoms persisted and I took more overdoses. When I explained that I felt distressed because of the way that I looked, I was dismissed. This increased my feelings of embarrassment and shame; I felt guilty for worrying so much about the way that I looked. The BDD increased, and my life revolved around the level of satisfaction I could achieve with the never-ending cycle of camouflage. I thought about my ugly appearance every moment of the day, and again became suicidal. I couldn't talk to family and friends about my feelings, because I was frightened that they would think that I was vain or mad. I couldn't understand how anyone could bear to look at me and not recoil in horror.

Then I saw an advertisement in the local paper for a facelift. Despite having these disturbing thoughts about my appearance, I hadn't really thought about plastic surgery before. But the more I researched it, the more I was convinced that it might just save my life. This seemed my last chance. I wanted surgery immediately. I went into hospital two weeks later and had a facelift and lower-eyelid surgery. I wasn't nervous or hesitant at all. This was an emergency. As the days passed and my face healed I could still see imperfections and my anxiety soared. I scrutinised every area of my face, and was convinced that I had made things worse and now it was all my own fault. How could I have been so stupid?

Within months I was back at the clinic, having injectable fillers that were painful, expensive, and only lasted a few months. The next year I went back to the hospital for more surgery. Afterwards I felt the same: disgusted by my appearance and horrified at what I had done. Despite all this, and because my BDD was so bad, I continued with injectable fillers and spent a fortune on various products over the next two years.

This unhealthy cycle of behaviour carried on until 2000. I didn't know where to turn. I was still seeing a psychiatrist and a psychologist, but my BDD remained undiagnosed. I survived another overdose, but it was followed by a spell of taking tablets day and night, because I could not stand the torturous thoughts. I decided to give cosmetic surgery another chance. After all, it might just work this time, and if it didn't I would end my life, which seemed inevitable anyway. Again, having made up my mind, I went to see a different surgeon and was operated on within the week for another facelift, chin tuck, eyebrow lift, and laser treatment. I cashed in my mortgage endowment policy to pay for the operations without a second thought.

I felt worse afterwards. It was around this time that I saw a TV programme about a girl who had a condition called BDD. I couldn't believe that I wasn't the only one who felt this way! I phoned the helpline and got information about BDD from OCD Action. Now, nearly seven years on, after years of excellent cognitive behavioural treatment, I understand that all the surgery I had was not helpful at all. It made my BDD worse, and far more dangerous. I have learned not to make demands on myself to look or be a certain way to be accepted. It is enough just to be me, and I am grateful for the life I am now living, which could so easily have been lost.

### *Niki

*"On school picture days, I would come home bawling."*

I was diagnosed with BDD when I was 19, a little over a year ago, and have spent my time since then trying to learn about this disorder. When I was first told I had it, I felt relieved that there was a name for what was wrong with me, but I also felt sad to have this illness. I remember when I was only nine years old I thought about cutting off my nose because it was too big. I was already tired of the snide remarks from friends and even strangers about how big it was.

When I was in junior high, my self-esteem issues went far beyond the average teenage angst. I couldn't bear to look in a mirror or have my picture taken. On school picture days I would come home bawling, because I knew that my nose would be posted everywhere. I wore a windbreaker with long sleeves so I could use the sleeve to cover up my face. It made me feel better. In high school I discovered my knack for humour. I made fun of myself before anyone else could get to me first. Deep inside the demon was ready to come bursting out. I was also addicted to painkillers.

After I was diagnosed with BDD along with panic disorder, I was put on an antidepressant that has saved me. No, it doesn't take away the thoughts about my nose or body; no, it doesn't give me hallucinations that I am a supermodel. But it helps me to think clearly, and not dwell on my physical problems. I know that no matter how many times people tell someone with BDD that they are beautiful, they still won't believe it. And what if you are absolutely the most gorgeous woman on the inside? Doesn't that matter too? That's what I try to tell myself each and every day. It's sort of my mantra now. I've noticed that once I stopped openly complaining about the way I looked, I began to receive more positive vibes from people. I am still not ready to be photographed but, hopefully, with time and therapy, I will make that giant step!

## What parents can do

Although there is no way to prevent BDD, it's advisable to get your child treatment as soon as symptoms appear. Likewise, teaching, encouraging, and modelling healthy attitudes about body image may help or, at least, keep it from getting worse. Exposure to realistic body types and providing a supportive environment can also decrease the severity of the symptoms.

Here's what one mother had to say about getting help after discovering her daughter's BDD.

## Chelsea's mum

*"As soon as I read about BDD online I knew this was what she had."*

Our world fell apart when Chelsea was in eighth grade. She clearly was having a very hard time, and she confided in me with her concerns. I was sure it was adolescent related, and I kept talking to her, figuring that I would eventually say those magic words that would make her all better. When that didn't happen, my husband and I found a local therapist for her to talk to. The sessions were not helping, but the therapist didn't have a diagnosis. As soon as I read about BDD online, I knew this was what she had.

I bought *The Broken Mirror* by Katharine Phillips and read it in a day. I read that patients need to be treated by professionals trained in helping those with BDD. When we were finally able to locate a BDD clinic, I cried on the phone with them, begging for their help because there weren't any other options. When she first started Cognitive Behaviour Therapy (CBT), she would cry most of the way home. It was hard work. Then things started to get better. After about four months, Chelsea was really improving and I agonised over what would happen to her when the therapy ended. By the end of the treatment she was doing amazingly well!

Things were pretty good for about nine months. Then I noticed that the rituals that she worked so hard in therapy to control were creeping back into our lives. She had a relapse that was so bad she was unable to function in school. We tried a number of other therapists in our area that were not specialists in BDD, because we could not find any that were. They couldn't help her.

She went on Lexapro for her depression. Her depression lifted, but the BDD wasn't getting any better. We went back to the BDD clinic to get specialised CBT, and she started practising her skills and began to get better again. Chelsea is in college now, and functioning quite well although she has her ups and downs. Our road has been long and exhausting, but my daughter would have no quality of life if it wasn't for the BDD treatment.

The most important advice I could give to a parent is to find experts to help your child. I also believe that CBT is amazingly effective if you and your child are willing to do the work. Chelsea continues to fight the thoughts that constantly invade her life. We are so incredibly proud of her.

## GETTING HELP

The idea of talking about your appearance-related concerns with your friends or family members may cause you further anxiety. You may worry that they will think you are vain or crazy. How could they possibly understand all the thoughts you are having? Remember, BDD is a *real* issue that affects other teens and young adults. You are not alone in this – nor are you crazy or vain, despite what you may be thinking or feeling. Help is out there for you.

Consider sharing your thoughts and concerns with a parent, teacher, coach, or another adult you trust. Sharing your thoughts and feelings with someone who can help you is the first step towards getting better. Once you decide on the best treatment option for you, you can get back to doing the things you love.

**Resources**

- The International OCD Foundation, iocdf.org
- The Body Dysmorphic Foundation, https://bddfoundation.org/
- Australian Psychological Society Tel. (03) 8662 3300 or 1800 333 497
- Mental Health Foundation of Australia (Victoria) Tel. (03) 9427 0406
- Lifeline (Australia) Tel. 13 11 14
- Butterfly Foundation https://butterfly.org.au/

## CHAPTER THREE

# BREAST WISHES

Our culture has long been obsessed with female breasts. Walk through any classical art museum, and you will see idealised portraits and sculptures of nude women dating from the dawn of time to present times. Despite, or perhaps because of, this fascination, research shows that the majority of women are unhappy with their breasts. A 2020 study of 18,541 women from 40 countries, discovered 48% wanted larger breasts, 23% wanted smaller breasts, and only 29% were satisfied with the size of their breasts. The average age of the women surveyed was 34.

This may explain why breast augmentation is the number one most requested procedure by women worldwide, with nearly two million surgeries performed annually – 30,000 in Australia alone – according to the Australian Society of Plastic Surgery (ASPS). Women who get augmented typically want a one- or two-cup-size increase. Those who want reductions typically go down one or two cup sizes. Most of the patients I see for breast surgery, whether larger or smaller, want it for themselves and how it makes them feel; rarely is it because partners encourage them to do so. In fact, many husbands who attend the consultations quite openly tell me that they would prefer their wives not to have surgery, but they are there to support them.

Fashion also plays a role in how women feel about their bodies, and from buxom Marilyn Monroe in the 1950s to the small-chested models of today, breast fashions evolve. But fashion is not always destiny, and whilst today's designers generally favor a petite chest, augmentation is three times as popular as reduction.

Aside from the desire for cosmetic improvements that lead women to get breast implants or reductions, congenital abnormalities are surprisingly common, and a source of significant distress to young women and their families. Broadly speaking, breast disorders can be thought of as underdevelopment, overdevelopment, or deformational (a change in either shape or size of the body), the most common developmental breast conditions that I see in my practice.

Timing is important if you – or your child – are considering surgery, as procedures to correct breast abnormalities in young people must balance growth and development as well as numerous psychological factors. Treatment goals need to be tailored to the individual, and rely on an accurate diagnosis to achieve the best cosmetic results. In other words, everything must be customised to each individual patient's needs and lifestyle, and what is perfect for one person may not be right for another's physical and psychological needs.

Before I discuss the different types of breast conditions and treatments, it's important to understand how female breasts develop in the first place:

## WHEN DOES BREAST DEVELOPMENT BEGIN?

It may surprise you to learn that the breast is actually a modified sweat gland that begins developing at about six weeks of life. Paired, proliferating stem cells migrate to form primitive mammary ridges – or the milk line – that extend on the front side of the fetus along the embryo from the armpits to the groin. The diagram on the next page shows the entire path the mammary ridge takes in women.

A healthy female breast, which is mostly fatty tissue, has 12 to 20 sections called lobes. Each lobe contains many smaller lobules, the gland that produces milk in nursing women. The lobes and ductal system develop at 20 weeks, and later the mammary pit forms at the origin of the mammary gland, contributing to the development of the nipple.

During development, portions along the mammary ridge shrink and atrophy as the fetus grows, except around the fourth rib, which sets the foundation for the primary mammary bud and future breast mound. This leaves behind only the primitive breast tissue on the chest wall, which then penetrates the underlying connective tissue during weeks 10 to 14. The connective tissue that now surrounds the breast ultimately forms the superficial fascial system of the breast and ligaments. Fascia is the connective tissue that holds organs, blood vessels, bones, nerve fibres and muscles in place – imagine the supports of a bridge. These structures become important when we discuss deformational conditions such as tuberous breasts (see page 69).

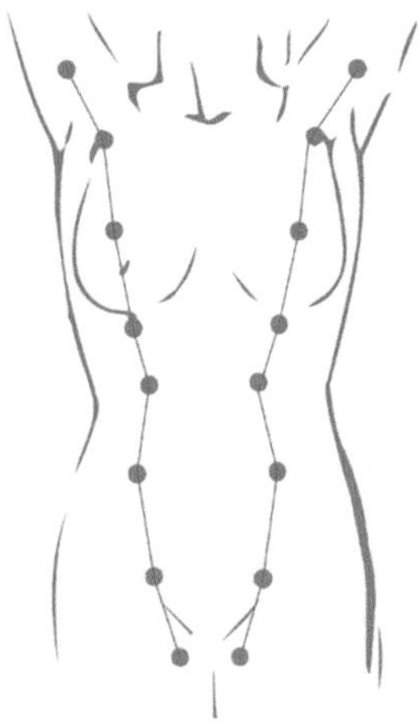

*Embryonic mammary ridges*

## WHAT BREAST CHANGES HAPPEN AT PUBERTY?

The first visible signs of breast development begin when a girl is a tween. Her ovaries start to produce and secrete estrogen, which causes fat in the connective tissue to collect. This is when breasts begin to grow along with the duct system. Teens may also notice the appearance of pubic and armpit hair. Once ovulation and menstruation begin, secretory glands form at the end of the milk ducts. The breasts and duct system continue to grow and mature along with the development of glands and lobules, and at the end of each lobule are tiny 'bulbs' that produce milk. These structures are linked by small tubes called ducts, which carry milk to the nipples. The size of the breasts increases as fat fills in the spaces between the lobes and ducts, and it's important for teens to understand that the rate at which breasts grow is different for each person. It is not unusual for some adolescents to have a growth spurt while others develop more slowly, and we know that sex hormones play a large role in breast development during puberty. You can see the different stages of breast development in the Tanner Scale below.

## THE TANNER SCALE OF THE FEMALE BREAST DEVELOPMENT

Stage 1 The breast is prepubertal, without appreciable breast tissue, and slight nipple elevation.

Stage 2 Begins with thelarche, which is the onset of secondary pubertal breast development. This stage marks the beginning of pubertal development. The nipple-areolar complex widens, and the breast and nipple become a small mound. The average age this occurs is around nine or ten.

Stage 3 The third stage is heralded with a further enlargement as the breast extends beyond the borders of the areola.

Stage 4 The nipple elevates above the breast contour as a secondary mound.

Stage 5 The breast achieves its final mature size and form.

## WHAT BREAST CHANGES OCCUR DURING THE MENSTRUAL CYCLE?

Each month women go through the hormonal changes that make up the normal menstrual cycle. When the hormone estrogen is produced by the ovaries in the first half of the menstrual cycle, it stimulates the growth of milk ducts in the breasts. The increasing level of estrogen leads to ovulation halfway through the cycle. Another hormone called progesterone takes over in the second half of the cycle, which stimulates the formation of the milk glands. These hormones are believed to be responsible for the cyclical changes that many women feel in their breasts right before their period starts. During this time it is normal to experience swelling, pain, and soreness in the breasts.

It's also normal for many women to feel changes in breast texture at this time. For some, breasts may feel lumpy. These textural changes are caused by enlarging glands in the breast that are preparing them for a possible pregnancy. If pregnancy does not happen, the breasts go back to normal size. Once menstruation starts, the cycle begins again.

## WHAT HAPPENS TO BREASTS DURING PREGNANCY AND MILK PRODUCTION?

Many healthcare providers believe breasts are not fully mature until a woman has given birth and produces milk. Breast changes are one of the earliest signs of pregnancy, a result of progesterone. In addition, the dark areas of skin around the nipples, the areolas, begin to swell, followed by the rapid swelling of the breasts themselves. Most pregnant women feel soreness on the sides of the breasts, as well as nipple tingling or pain due to the growth of the milk duct system and formation of many more lobules.

By the fifth or sixth month of pregnancy, the breasts are fully capable of producing milk. As in puberty, estrogen controls the growth of the ducts, and progesterone controls the growth of the glandular buds. Other hormones play vital roles in milk production, including follicle-stimulating hormone (FSH), luteinizing hormone (LH), prolactin, oxytocin, and human placental lactogen (HPL). Meanwhile other physical changes are taking place: the blood vessels in the breast become more visible and the areola gets larger and darker. All of these changes are a preparation for breastfeeding after birth.

However, these are some of the things that can go wrong, and potential treatments:

## POLYTHELIA OR EXTRA NIPPLES

What do Harry Styles, Mark Wahlberg and Tilda Swinton have in common? Aside from being famous, all have extra nipples – a common congenital

## OXYTOCIN OR THE LOVE HORMONE

Oxytocin is sometimes called the love or cuddle hormone, because it's released by the brain when people snuggle up or socialise. It is a particularly important hormone for women during motherhood, and said to create a bond between a mother and infant while nursing. Playing with a pet can also cause an oxytocin spike, according to a 2009 study published in the journal *Hormones and Behaviour*.

abnormality that affects both women and men. Supernumerary nipples can appear anywhere along the mammary path and, according to the Genetic and Rare Diseases Information Center (GARD), approximately 200,000 Americans have extra nipples. An Israeli study found one in 40 babies are born with supernumerary nipples, most commonly found below the breast and above the lower abdominal skin. They appear on both sides of the body in 50% of the cases. Patients who come to me with extra nipples are frequently embarrassed by this. Fortunately, the treatment is a straightforward surgical removal of the extra nipple.

## GIGANTOMASTIA/JUVENILE HYPERTROPHY OR EXTREMELY LARGE BREASTS

Gigantomastia is a rare condition that causes excessive growth of the female breasts. There are several names for this condition in young people, including juvenile hypertrophy or virginal mammary hypertrophy, which typically occurs in late childhood and early adolescence. Although the exact cause of this sudden and rapid breast growth is unknown, it is thought to be caused by an excess of local estrogen production, abnormal estrogen receptor sensitivity, and the presence of an estrogen-like substance.

### *Treatment for gigantomastia*

The mainstay for treatment is surgery to raise and reshape and reduce large breasts. Although it is prudent to wait approximately one year after breast growth has ended before having breast reduction surgery, highly symptomatic patients may require an early reduction procedure. I inform all of my patients that they will likely require a second breast reduction later in their life.

### *What is involved in a breast reduction?*

The goal of a breast reduction is exactly that: to reduce the size of the skin and breast tissue. The procedure removes excess fat, glandular tissue, and skin from the breast, leaving patients with a breast size that is in proportion with their body, and alleviating the discomfort. The surgery takes approximately two hours, and the results are physically and psychologically transformative.

To get the best results, the breast needs to be lifted and also reshaped – reducing the size of the breast without lifting and reshaping is undesirable. When planning a reduction the surgeon must consider the patient's weight, age, goals, degree of sagginess, and the overall skin quality. Surgeons use a combination of various procedures, depending on the patient's needs and goals. All procedures, except for liposuction and breast reduction with a nipple graft, require maintaining a blood supply to the nipple-areola complex. Liposuction, which is slimming and reshaping areas of the body by removing excess fat, is rarely performed, but ideally suited for treating macromastia, a condition in which the breast tissue contains a high proportion of fatty tissue and the breast has good shape and skin elasticity. Additionally, liposuction is not a good choice in the young patient who typically has very dense and fibrous breast tissue with little fat.

Your surgeon has four major considerations when planning a breast reduction:

1. What incisions to use
2. How much breast tissue needs resection
3. How to reshape the breast
4. How to manage excess skin.

Remember that the goal of breast reduction is not only to reduce the breast volume, but also to reposition and reshape the breast.

## WILL THERE BE SCARRING AFTER A BREAST REDUCTION?

Like any surgery, breast reductions will leave some scars. The extent of the scarring, however, depends on the type of procedure – that is to say, shorter-scar versus larger-scar techniques (see the different techniques

## BIG-BREASTED WOMAN GETS FIRST REDUCTION PROCEDURE

The first breast reduction procedure on record was performed in 1669 by British physician Dr. William Darston, who wrote about his "big breasted" patient.

Although gigantomastia is noncancerous, having extremely large breasts can be physically and emotionally debilitating. Many of the patients who come to me with oversized breasts complain of severe back, shoulder and neck pain, poor posture, redness or itching under the breasts, and general breast pain. Others are troubled by the unwanted attention of peers and strangers. In my experience, the self-consciousness and emotional discomfort many of my patients with large, pendulous breasts feel is just as important as the physical discomfort and pain they can cause.

below). Most scars are located on the lower half of the breast below the nipple, which may be covered with a bra or swimsuit. Be sure to talk to your doctor about which technique is best for you, and post-operative care.

### *Shorter-scar technique*

The shorter-scar technique in breast reduction surgery involves smaller incisions. This method is used for patients with sagging breasts who want a minimal-to-moderate reduction in breast size. These patients usually want to go down a cup size. Shorter-scar techniques aren't as effective for larger breast reductions.

### *Vertical reduction*

Also called a lollipop reduction, this technique involves two incisions. The first is made around the areola, and the other is made from the bottom of the areola down toward the underlying breast crease. Once the incisions are made, your surgeon will remove tissue, fat, and excess skin before reshaping the breast to a smaller size. Because these incisions are smaller, the scarring is condensed to a small area of the breast.

### *Larger-scar technique (anchor reduction)*

As the name suggests, larger-scar techniques involve more incisions and produce larger areas of scarring. This technique involves three incisions:

- One between the areola and crease under the breast
- Another around the areola
- A final incision horizontally beneath the breast along the crease.

The larger-scar technique is used for what's called the inverted-T or anchor breast reduction. People best suited for this procedure have significant asymmetry or sagging, and your surgeon may also suggest an anchor reduction if you want to go down a few cup sizes or more. Although more extensive, the larger-scar technique only involves one additional incision underneath the breasts.

## IS IT POSSIBLE TO BREASTFEED AFTER A REDUCTION?

Women considering breast reduction prior to having children often ask about breast feeding following surgery. The good news for patients who want to nurse is that studies have shown that breast reduction surgery does not interfere with a woman's ability to breastfeed.

In one 2007 study published in the *Journal of the American Society of Plastic Surgery*, researchers compared 164 women who nursed after breast reduction surgery with 151 women of similar weight and age who had not had the procedure. They found 62% in the non-surgical group successfully breastfed, as did 63% who had had the operation – a negligible difference. The remainder supplemented with formula.

## BREAST AMPUTATION AND FREE NIPPLE GRAFT

Lastly, for extremely large (2000g) reductions and breasts with very low nipples, a breast amputation with a free nipple graft is favoured. In these patients, an amputation is performed based on the anchor skin pattern, and the nipple is removed and repositioned as a graft on the breast mound. Patients who have this technique cannot breastfeed after surgery, as the ducts are not reestablished because the nipple is only replaced for aesthetic enhancement rather than functional benefit.

## WILL THERE BE NIPPLE SENSATION AFTER BREAST REDUCTION?

There is no definitive answer to this question. Nipple sensation can either permanently decrease, increase, or not change after surgery, but the nerve supply to the nipples comes out from around the fourth rib and is rarely sacrificed or damaged during the operation. Studies report permanent loss of nipple sensation in approximately 2–5% of patients, but, interestingly, in some patients the nipple sensation actually improves because the weight and stretch of the nerve are taken away after the removal of breast tissue.

Early changes in sensation are often temporary with full sensation returning in 6–12 months.

## CAN I CHOOSE MY CUP SIZE AFTER A BREAST REDUCTION?

Most women with gigantomastia do not wear the correct bra size. There are a multitude of reasons for this, including social stigma associated with bra size, lack of knowledge about what constitutes a well-fitted bra, and, more importantly, the fact that most bras don't fit large or uneven breasts. Nonetheless, patients use cup size as the most objective way of communicating their ultimate goals to their surgeon, and doctors must acknowledge the limitations of only using cup size as the defining factor for a patient's desires. Talk to your surgeon about your ideal cup size before having any procedure, and keep an open mind. I ask my patients about their desired cup size, and to bring in photos of breasts in sizes and shapes that they are happy with. This gives me an idea of how much I need to reduce their breasts to achieve those results.

When planning a breast reduction, surgeons must calculate how many grams of breast tissue need to be removed to get the desired cup size. The medical literature on bra cup size and volume is relatively sparse, which led me to conduct a scientific study in 2017 that explored the issue. The aim of this study, which was published in *Plastic and Reconstructive Surgery*, was to identify the volume increase between cup sizes in three popular brands of bra, and samples of bra cup sizes from B through E, all with an Australian size 12 band equivalent to a US size 34 and an international size 75, were analysed for their volume capacity. I found a considerable variation in volume capacity within the same bra cup size of the different brands tested, and also inconsistencies within the same manufacturer, with no fixed volume increase between cup sizes. In other words, the volume difference from B cup to C cup is not the same incremental increase as from C cup to D cup.

## VOLUME CAPACITY OF EACH BRA CUP SIZE

The chart below gives the ratio of cup size to grams of breast tissue. As you will see, our study found that the volume of breast tissue varies by the manufacturer's cup size.

| Bra brand and cup size | Mean volume of cup (cc) |
|---|---|
| Brand 1 | |
| 12B | 433 |
| 12C | 632 |
| 12D | 728 |
| 12DD | 908 |
| 12E | 1040 |
| Brand 2 | |
| 12B | 491 |
| 12C | 576 |
| 12D | 704 |
| 12DD | 797 |
| 12E | 924 |
| Brand 3 | |
| 12B | 467 |
| 12C | 697 |
| 12D | 834 |
| 12DD | 920 |
| 12E | 1053 |

The study scientifically confirmed two key points that patients and plastic surgeons have known intuitively for years: (1) There is no one standard for cup sizes and volume in the bra manufacturing industry; and (2) One should not aim for a desired cup size, but rather a look. If a patient requests a certain bra cup size the physician should estimate based on the fact that 130–150cc equals one cup size.

## *Sophie, 24, Sydney

When I turned 14, my breasts went from average to a D/DD. By the time I was 16, they had jumped two or three sizes to an E/G cup. They were huge! I've got quite a small frame, so my breasts made me look five kilos bigger than I was. My mum had very large breasts and had also had a reduction, so it's definitely genetic. In the beginning, I had a love-hate relationship with my breasts. I loved them because they made me stick out from the crowd – literally. I was "Sophie, the girl with big boobs", and I enjoyed the attention. Many of my friends would tell me they wished theirs were bigger. I don't think they were actually envious of *my* big boobs, but young girls going through puberty want to know they're going to get bigger at some point.

I hated them because they were an obstacle in life. I had trouble shopping for clothing, exercising, sleeping, and showering. I was also a dancer from the age of three, and they were becoming more and more of a nightmare. I had to wear two sports bras, and sometimes strap them down with sports tape. I had the same issues in sports class – running was nearly impossible with big boobs. Shopping for bikinis was especially hard because the nice swimsuits and lacy bras never seemed to support me. Mine looked like nana bras – those big, ugly support things that only come in skin colour. I would sleep in my bra – mostly on my side, because when I lay on my back I would feel a bit squashed and suffocated. It was so hard to find clothes that were flattering to my figure and didn't just hang off me to fit my breasts.

I would get a lot of judgemental looks, and hear whispers about what I wore if too much of my breasts were revealed in an outfit, most of the time from other girls. There was this strange mentality that if a teenage girl has big boobs, she had to be a skank. Groups of teenage boys would surround me chanting "tits out for the boys" to get me to flash my breasts. The most slut-shaming happened on Facebook and Instagram from keyboard warriors who would say disgusting sexual things about my breasts. I didn't have any serious relationships in high school, which I'm fairly sure was due to my having super large breasts.

I also had lots of back problems. Anytime I wasn't wearing a bra my back would hurt. I would always shower in a bikini, especially when washing my hair, to avoid backache. I would also get a strong stabbing pain in my chest whenever I'd do vigorous exercise. I went to the doctor about it, and she diagnosed pectoral girdle dysfunction. Because my breasts were so large, the muscles contracted and spasmed to support my upper body, which put pressure on my ribs and chest.

That's when I decided to get a breast reduction. My mum was really eager for me to get it, mainly because she knew that I would be happier after it. I wasn't nervous from a medical perspective, but I was worried that I wouldn't feel like me afterwards. I still wanted big boobs, just not too big, which is silly but probably a common request when women have breast reductions. I wanted to go to a D/DD, but my mum and Dr Moradi convinced me to go to a C.

I had the surgery when I was 17, and I remember Dr. Moradi telling me that it was the largest surgery he had ever done and on his youngest patient! The surgery took about six hours, and the recovery was painful – it took several months before I could go back to normal daily life. Medication helped with the pain. I wasn't able to lift my arms above 45 degrees, and I had to wear maternity bras. When I first woke up after surgery there was a lot of swelling, and my breasts were stitched down into place. My chest was so flat that I cried out of sadness, but after a few months the swelling went down and my breasts are now C/D and perfect for my body shape and size!

I love my new breasts. One of my best girlfriends got hers reduced last year, and she also says it was the best decision ever. I can now go running – I rarely went running before due to the pain – swim, play tennis, and do Pilates without having to wear an extra sports bra or strapping. If you have large breasts and they don't cause you any grief, then embrace them and enjoy them through life! But if you aren't happy with them or experience any of the difficulties I had with mine, I can't recommend a reduction highly enough. I'm currently in graduate school, and I'm in a long-term relationship. The operation was life-changing!

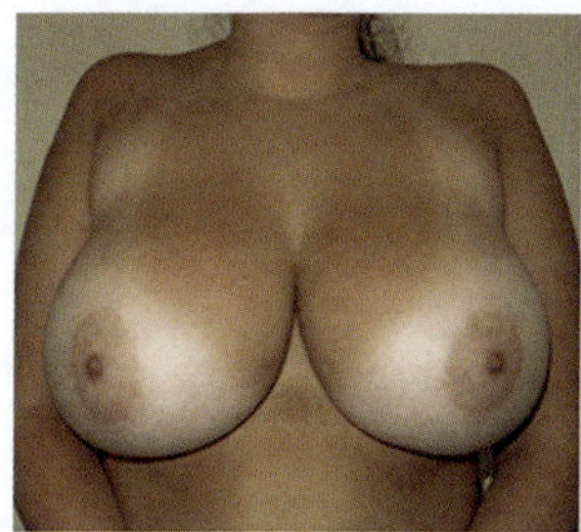
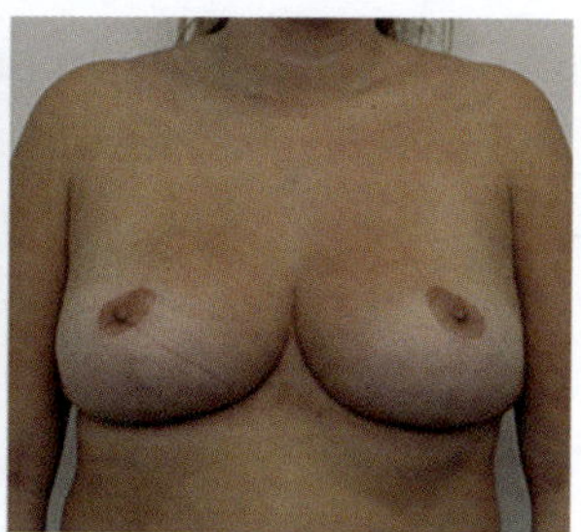

## TUBEROUS/TUBULAR BREASTS

When one breast is larger than the other, it is known as tuberous or tubular, named for the resemblance to the shape of a tuberous plant root. This is a rare condition that affects young women during puberty in either one or both breasts. The deformity is characterised by a constricting ring at the base of the breast, which leads to deficient horizontal and vertical development. Having tuberous breasts makes wearing a bra nearly impossible, because one cup would be an A and the other a D. Other characteristics of tuberous breasts include:

- Deficiency in the width of the breast
- Elevated inframammary breast fold

- Short nipple-to-crease distance due to the deficient breast tissue in the lower half of the breast
- Herniation of the breast tissue through the areola resulting in enlarged areolar
- Underdeveloped breast tissue
- Asymmetry.

### *What causes tuberous breasts?*

While it is not known what causes tuberous breasts, there are several theories. Since the breast tissue comes from the ectodermis, the stem cells that give rise to the skin, the breast develops as these cells penetrate the deeper soft tissue layer called the mesoderm. During this invagination process, the breast is contained within a fascial envelope called the superficial fascia, and the outer and inner lawyers of the fascia surround the entirety of the breast tissue like a glove. The deep layer of the superficial fascia is penetrated by fibrous attachments that join the two layers of the superficial fascia, and extend to the skin and the muscle layer. Tuberous breasts develop when the outer layer of the superficial fascia is absent in the area underneath the areola, which creates herniation of the breast tissue through the areolar. There is also a constricting ring at the lower aspect of the breast that restricts and inhibits the normal development of breast growth, and this constricting ring of fibrous tissue does not allow the developing breast tissue to expand and develop during puberty.

### *Treatment for tuberous breasts*

Surgery for tuberous breasts is often performed in stages, with two or three procedures done three to six months apart. The extent of the correction depends on the deformity that needs to be addressed to create symmetry, and I tell my patients that their breasts will look like sisters, not identical twins, as it is impossible to make the breasts look exactly the same. The following procedures are considered when operating on tuberous breast patients to achieve the best possible results:

- Implants and/or fat grafting to augment the deficient volume
- Breast lift to reshape and lift the breast tissue
- Areola reduction to reduce and support the nipple areolar complex.

## *Alice, 22, Sydney

"I first noticed my breasts were different sizes when I was 12. At that time, there was just a small size difference, so I brushed it off and continued to be a kid with no worries. As the years went on, my left breast grew to a solid D cup while my right stayed completely flat. I was in total denial back then, telling myself it's not that bad – everyone has different sized boobs. Looking back, I feel sorry for that girl trying to justify her appearance. I didn't do or say anything about it until I was 16. After that, my mum, my grandmother, and my best friend were the only people who knew about my abnormality.

At first, mum and grandmother thought I was overreacting and being dramatic. They tried to convince me that I was being superficial and that I only wanted an excuse for plastic surgery. I remember arguing with my grandmother for a solid hour, telling her that I wasn't crazy and that this wasn't normal! I became so angry, I finally lifted up my shirt and bra to show her. She was speechless. From that day on until my surgeries, she would sew padding into the right side of my clothing so my abnormality wouldn't be so noticeable, but even with the padding I didn't feel confident, and some of my friends would ask me why my boobs looked so funny.

When I turned 18, my gran had to double the padding to create a symmetrical shape no matter what outfit I was wearing. I wore a padded bra while I slept! Going to the beach was impossible for me, because it was just a panic attack waiting to happen. I couldn't wear bikinis or a one-piece. I felt like I couldn't hide my breast sizes with so little support. And forget about spaghetti straps or those strapless tops that looked amazing on all the other girls. Sometimes I covered myself up from head to toe in loose, unfitted clothing because I felt like everyone was judging me. Having tuberous breasts isn't physically painful, but I became really depressed. I wouldn't go shopping or go out with friends, because I always felt self-conscious and unfeminine. I wouldn't go out – period.

My mum encouraged me to ask a gynecologist about my breasts. He had no idea what was wrong with me, but told me I should wait until I was done with puberty before seeking any medical advice. I was 20 when I saw Dr. Moradi, and at my first consultation, he asked me "What do you want to achieve?" I told him three things: the symmetry of both breasts, natural-looking breasts, and quality that would last for years. I didn't want to come back in a few years to get things redone. He really listened and told me about everything I should consider. He explained that I needed three surgeries and why they were necessary.

I had three surgeries over a 10-month period. I remember downloading a calendar countdown app and jumping for joy the day of my first procedure. Dr. Moradi's goal was to make the right breast skin stretch as much as possible by implanting an expander (a pouch that would stretch the skin over the next three months). Then he performed a breast lift on the left side. He went a step further by placing the expander into the right side. The pain was a solid 9/10. It felt like someone had punched me in the centre of my chest. I was given muscle relaxers and pain meds. Recovery took two months.

I was really nervous before my second surgery. I anticipated the pain I had felt after the first surgery, but I was beyond delighted to find that there was just a mild pain. This time Dr. Moradi inserted the implants and performed another lift on the left breast because the skin had stretched more than initially thought. He took some fat from my belly and injected it into the breast to create an even cleavage and give a more natural look and feel to the breast. Recovery time this round was two to three weeks.

By the third surgery, I was a pro. I walked in and walked out without any of my pain meds. This was an optional surgery. Dr Moradi told me we could finish after the second surgery, but he would prefer to fix up and tighten a few things to make the transformation more permanent. He performed a small lift on the left breast and injected further fat into both breasts. The pain was almost non-existent and the recovery was quick.

After the first surgery, I immediately saw the difference in my breast shape, size and weight. I got home from the hospital and threw away my padding. After the second surgery I made it a point to go get measured for bras. I became a 12E cup (34DD US/34E UK). After my final procedure I went out for the first time ever and bought a bikini. I took my best friend with me, and it was such an amazing and freeing experience. No anxiety, no secrets, and no more worries about covering up. The next day I came home from the beach with the most amazing tan lines and glow. I never wanted to cover up again! I felt like a confident woman for the first time in my life.

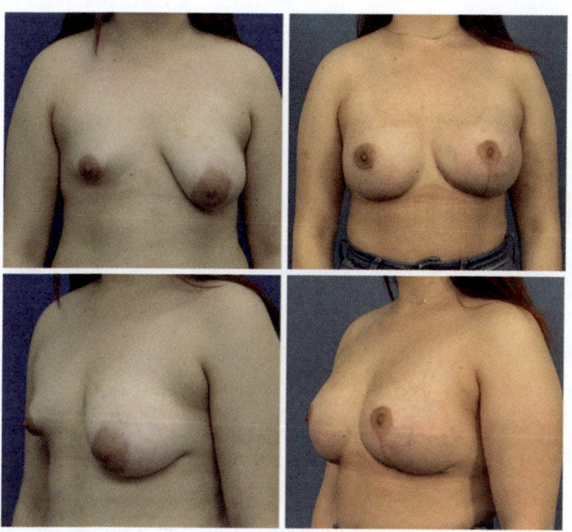

*Alice before and after*

My advice for anyone who has tuberous breasts like I did is to surround yourself with the right support group. Keep it small. These are the people who will give you the support you will need during your transformation.

If you are looking into plastic surgery, find the right surgeon for you. Dr Moradi was the right surgeon for me because he understood the results I wanted. He took that time to listen, and explained in detail what he wanted to do and why he felt it was the best approach in the long run. Don't be ashamed if you do want to have plastic surgery. Do the surgery only for *yourself*. Don't do it because you want to impress someone.

I'm happy to say that I have been dating since my last surgery. My confidence and all-around personality have really opened up, which has made it possible for me to go out, have fun and meet people. Now I'm carefree!

## AMASTIA

The condition where breast tissue fails to develop within the embryonic mammary ridge is called amastia. While rare, the earliest record of amastia appears in the Bible: "We have a little sister, and she hath no breasts" (Song of Solomon VIII:8). The typical treatment for amastia is a combination of breast reconstruction and psychological counselling.

## POLYMASTIA OR EXTRA BREASTS

Polymastia is the development of excess breast tissue with or without the presence of a nipple. This typically develops along the mammary ridge after hormonal stimulation. Incomplete absorption of the mammary ridge anywhere along this line produces excess breast tissue (i.e. an additional breast). The condition occurs in about 2–6% of females and 1–3% of males.

An extreme case recorded in 1827 occurred in Thérèse Ventre of Marseille, France, who had a fully formed third breast on her left thigh. According to an article published in *American Surgeon*, this breast began to produce milk after she had given birth. "It was offered to her infant who took it willingly," her doctor was quoted as saying. Ventre never had the additional breast removed, and she reportedly nursed five children from all three of her breasts.

## PECTUS EXCAVATUM OR SHALLOW CHEST

Pectus excavatum is a developmental deformity that produces a concave appearance in the central chest wall. It's the most common congenital chest wall abnormality, and the cause is unknown. Although no specific genetic defect has been linked to this, familial recurrence is reported in 35% of cases. Pectus excavatum occurs in one in 300–400 live births, with boys affected three times more often than girls. The condition is often noticed soon after birth, with more than 90% of cases diagnosed within the first year. The condition typically worsens at the onset of adolescence (12–14 years), and continues into the teenage years.

### *Treatment for shallow chest*

The severity of the deformity dictates how aggressive you need to be in treating the condition. Generally speaking, there are two approaches to treating pectus excavatum. First, incisions are made under the breast crease, after which the muscles of the chest wall along with the affected sternum are removed, reshaped, moulded and replaced in the chest wall. The second option involves placement of a curved Nuss bar behind the bone, which is designed to push the sternum forward, allowing the remodeling of chest wall cartilage and bone. The bar is typically left in place for two years, and removed in a second operation.

## PECTUS CARINATUM OR PIGEON CHEST

Pectus carinatum, also known as pigeon chest or raised chest, is a condition where the breastbone and ribs protrude. It occurs approximately 10 times less often than pectus excavatum, and makes up 5–7% of congenital chest wall deformities.

### *Treatment for pigeon chest*

I tell patients who come to me to correct this condition that the process is similar to building a house. As a surgeon, I am both architect and builder, and we must start with a parcel of land as the foundation, the land being the patient's chest wall. Any asymmetries in the chest wall must be accurately diagnosed and addressed when considering breast aesthetics, and surgery to correct chest wall deformities usually involves remodelling of the cartilage and bony structures.

## POLAND SYNDROME

Poland syndrome is a rare developmental disorder characterised by the absence of chest wall muscles on one side of the body, and abnormally short, webbed fingers of the hand on the same side. Those with the condition are typically missing the pectoralis minor, which is the thin, triangular muscle of the upper chest wall, and the breastbone portion of the pectoralis major, the large, fanlike muscle that covers most of the upper front part of the chest. The full spectrum of the condition may also mean the absence of multiple ribs along with the chest wall depression, the absence of breasts or armpit hair, and an underdeveloped or missing nipple-areola complex.

The disorder was named after Alfred Poland, who first reported the condition in 1841 after dissecting a cadaver while studying anatomy at Guy's Hospital in London. I worked at Guy's more than a century and a half later, and recall seeing the plaque commemorating his findings. Sadly, my time there did not yield any groundbreaking discoveries, although I did meet my wife, and it was during this rotation that my then mentor, a paediatric cardiac surgeon named David Anderson, advised me to pursue a career in plastic surgery.

Poland syndrome occurs in one out of every 20,000–30,000 live births. It affects more men than women (3:1), and is found on the right side of the body in 75% of the cases. The exact cause is unknown, but it is thought to result from a disruption of the blood supply to the chest wall and arms during the sixth to seventh week of gestation. Another hypothesis is that it is a disruption of the mesodermal or middle layer of the embryonic tissue that gives rise to the chest wall muscles. In the embryology of the breast, the ectodermal breast tissue divides down and incorporates into the mesodermal soft tissue stem cells. Without soft tissue stem cells, the breast will not develop.

### *Treatment for Poland syndrome*

The treatment depends on the patient's specific symptoms, and may require a team of specialists, including a genetic counsellor. Plastic surgery is performed to rebuild the chest wall and to graft ribs into their proper places. In women, plastic surgery procedures can be used to construct a breast mound, and in some cases, surgery will help correct skeletal abnormalities affecting other areas of the body such as the hands. Physical therapy may also be prescribed to help improve any motion limitations.

## SOME OTHER INSIGHTS

It's important to remember that teens should reach full emotional and physical maturity before having surgery for many of the above conditions, and the same goes for rhinoplasty/nose jobs. However, there are exceptions to this rule. For example, if a teen has grossly asymmetric or extremely large breasts at the age of 15 that are causing both emotional and physical issues, then waiting until she is older is unnecessary as the deformity will not correct itself. Nor will diet, exercise or lifestyle changes. Sometimes the only option is surgery, and as you can see in Sophia's and Alice's stories, the emotional and psychological turmoil their breast conditions caused them was real and ever-present. Delaying treatment only prolonged their anguish.

A paediatrician and general practitioner can offer advice to some extent about the psychological suitability of surgery, but I have found their knowledge of adolescent breast deformities and available treatment options to be lacking and, at times, detrimental to the teens' well-being. For example, I recently saw a 15-year-old patient with severe tuberous deformity whose GP said not to worry about it until she turned 18, and that "she will grow into her body." I don't mean any disrespect to these physicians as they provide an invaluable service to the community, but such highly specialised conditions require early consultations with specialists.

Whilst social media and online forums have their pitfalls, I also find, when used properly, they are an excellent source of information that empowers patients. The ease of access to content allows most of my patients to learn about their condition and treatment before they visit me, bypassing the traditional referral pathway from their local GP.

When it comes to breast procedures, parents and doctors should also rule out any psychiatric issues, such as BDD. Patients should speak to their doctor one-on-one so they can feel comfortable about discussing issues they might not tell their parents about. It's equally important to talk about needs and expectations with family present to assess the degree of support. I always ask my patients to tell me why they want the surgery, so I can make sure that their expectations are realistic, and they understand potential risks. Before any surgery, you should consider how you would handle a complication should it arise or, in a more likely scenario, when everything goes as planned but the results just aren't exactly as you had imagined. For me, there is no greater reward than sending a patient home with a newfound self-confidence after a successful procedure that makes them feel normal.

## CHAPTER FOUR

# FACE VALUES

Like it or not, a pretty face, especially for women, has many advantages. The more attractive you are, the easier it is to get a job, and the more money you will make. Beautiful people, women and men alike, are also thought to be smarter and friendlier than less attractive people. It's not fair, but it's true – and research backs this up.

In one study, nearly 300 university students were asked to view photographs of young women's faces that varied in attractiveness. After looking at each photo, the students answered questions such as how likely she was to be popular, friendly, helpful, kind, or smart. Both men and women ranked people with unappealing faces as less intelligent, less sociable, and less likely to help others. Moderately attractive people got similar rankings to very beautiful people for everything except sociability. The researchers repeated the experiment with children aged seven to nine, and got the same results.

Scientists suspect this may be because unattractive faces look less like a normal or average face, and since the face is what we notice initially when meeting someone, it's an important factor for first impressions. Being aware of these biases can help us avoid making snap judgments about people based on appearance, and keep us from discriminating against those who are less attractive. Even though I'm in the business of making people look good, I agree with what the famously beautiful actress Audrey Hepburn once said: "True beauty in a woman is reflected in her soul. It's the caring that she lovingly gives, the passion that she shows..."

## THE BEAUTY IDEAL

When it comes to a beautiful face, it's all about symmetry. Attractive faces have full lips, a high forehead, small chin, small nose, short, narrow jaw, high cheekbones, clear, smooth skin, and wide-set eyes. Of course, one can still be attractive without having all these characteristics, but this is what is considered conventionally beautiful. Artists and researchers have actually calculated some of these ideal proportions, and mathematically quantified this harmony. Arthur Swift, a board-certified plastic surgeon who teaches at McGill University in Canada, created the Golden Ratio theory, which is a mathematical relationship found in beautiful things. You can see it in architecture, music, and famous works of art, such as the Venus de Milo, a Stradivarius violin, and Notre-Dame Cathedral.

The same ratio can be applied to the human face, although if you're not a model or movie star, it is difficult to achieve this universal mathematical ideal. But what we plastic surgeons strive for is balance. If you look in the mirror or one of the facial symmetry apps on your phone, you may notice differences and imbalances when one side of the face is compared to the other. What cosmetic surgery can create or recreate is this facial balance and harmony. The following are some of the more common procedures that help achieve facial symmetry:

## RHINOPLASTY OR NOSE JOB

Getting a nose job, which doctors call rhinoplasty, is the most common cosmetic surgery in patients of 18 or younger according to ASPS, with a total of 821,890 procedures performed annually worldwide. When done correctly by an experienced surgeon, rhinoplasty can give you that sought-after facial balance. The following are common reasons to consider this procedure:

- The nose is too large or too small
- The nose does not seem to fit with the rest of the face
- The nose is crooked, misshapen, or out of alignment
- A nasal blockage causes breathing problems
- There is a birth defect
- Negative self-image or self-esteem.

Rhinoplasty can also be done to change how you look or for medical reasons. For example, some people may need surgery to repair a problem with the cartilage that divides one nostril from the other: a deviated septum. Fixing a deviated septum or septoplasty can help a patient breathe more easily.

## WHEN CAN TEENS HAVE A RHINOPLASTY?

Teens should not have a rhinoplasty until their nose has reached its adult size. This normally happens at about 15 or 16 for girls. The age of consent for a nose job in Australia is 18, or younger with parental consent, psychological evaluation and clearance.

### *The consultation*

The surgeon will examine the inside and outside of the nose. Bones, cartilage, and breathing are evaluated. Photos of all sides of the face are taken and viewed in order to design a surgical plan. During the consultation, I routinely use 3D Vectra technology, which is a software program that allows me to capture a 3D image of the patient's face. I can then simulate the changes I plan on making during surgery with the likely outcomes. Check out my YouTube channel https://youtu.be/dzU1o7PwHP8 where I explain how this works. With the rise of app-based technologies, many of my patients have already downloaded and used similar apps to show the results they are after. I find this extremely helpful during the consultation process, as patients take control of their surgical journey, and this allows me to understand their goals.

### *What are the risks?*

The risks of rhinoplasty include:

- Scarring
- Post-operative breathing issues
- Unfavourable cosmetic outcomes
- Bleeding
- Infection

- Swelling
- Expectations not met.

Honest communication between the patient, parents, and surgeon is crucial to the success of the operation. It's important to understand that the final results with a rhinoplasty can take over a year. The reason for this is the amount of swelling in the skin and soft tissues around the nose. As with any procedure, teens and their parents should discuss all of the risks and benefits with the surgeon. I often tell patients that they can't have a particular type of nose – for example, if they have a large thick-skinned ethnic nose, they will never get a small, cute button nose. The skin canvas and bone structure won't allow it.

I like to take ample time to talk with my patients before surgery. When the patient is a teen, I want to make sure she is mature enough to handle the procedure, that she is doing it for the correct reasons, and that she has realistic expectations about the results. Thinking that changing your nose will change your whole life, or make you more popular is not realistic. The goal should always be improvement, not perfection.

### *Will there be scarring?*

Below are two types of nose surgery incisions:

1. *Open rhinoplasty.* An open rhinoplasty is performed by creating a small incision on the underside of the nose between the nostrils in a fairly Z-shaped pattern. This allows for more precise, accurate changes to be made to the shape of the nose. I use this technique in the majority of patients, especially if they want to make the nose smaller and refine the tip
2. *Closed rhinoplasty.* Incisions are made inside the nasal passages. Because these incisions are hidden, they are invisible after surgery. I only use this technique if patients wish to have a hump removed from their nasal dorsum or want the nose straightened.

### *Recovery*

It takes roughly six weeks for the bones in the nose to heal following surgery. During this time, you should avoid strenuous exercise. Even movements that seem harmless like stretching, lifting, or bending can increase nasal swelling. Pain will usually last for between 36 to 72 hours, but longer if the nose is touched or bumped. The nose may remain tender or sensitive to touch, however, for up to three months. As it takes a long time to get your final results, patients need to trust the process and be patient. As a rough guide, I tell them the upper two-thirds of the nose takes about six to eight weeks to get its final shape, but the tip can take up to a year.

## OTOPLASTY OR EAR SURGERY, EAR PINNING

Did you know that more people are born with prominent ears than any other head and neck anomaly? Approximately 15–20% of newborns present with misshapen ears that do not self-correct. Whilst there are many different ear abnormalities, I concentrate on prominent ear deformity. Prominent ears are relatively common, with an incidence of about 5%. It is inherited as an autosomal dominant trait, and commonly caused by a combination of three defects:

1. Underdevelopment of antihelical folding
2. Overdevelopment of the conchal wall
3. Protrusion of the ear away from the skull.

Although these deformities have no health consequences, numerous studies show the psychological distress, emotional trauma, and behavioural problems protruding ears can inflict on children, namely schoolyard bullying. Otoplasty is a cosmetic procedure that alters the size, position, or proportion of the ears. If the ears stick out, pinning surgery can be performed to flatten them against the head. If one ear is positioned higher than the other, ear repositioning can create that sought-after symmetry.

Oversized ears can be addressed alone or in conjunction with other ear issues. Like rhinoplasty, ear reshaping surgery helps boost self-confidence, especially in children, tweens, and teens. The following are common reasons for getting these procedures:

- Ears are overly large or small
- Ears are disproportionate to the head or oddly placed
- Ears protrude or stick out prominently
- An injury has negatively impacted the shape or positioning of the ears
- Negative self-esteem or self-image.

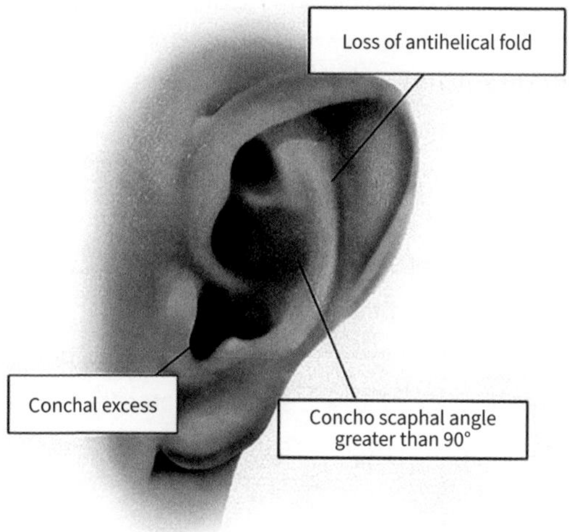


*Anatomy of the ear*

The ear is a complex composite of cartilage and skin with many intricate involutions and folds. There are five critical elements – concha, helix, antihelix, tragus, and lobule – and parts of lesser importance, including the antitragus, intertragic notch, and Darwin's tubercle. The anatomical divisions of the ear are developed at birth, with their origins based on the first (mandibular) and second (hyoid) branchial arches. The hyoid arch is the predominant contributor leading to the formation of the helix, scapha, antihelix, concha, antitragus, and lobule, whereas the mandibular arch only contributes to the tragus and helical crus.

The ear attains approximately 85% of its adult size by the age of three. Ear width reaches its mature size in boys of seven and in girls of six. Ear length matures in boys when they are 13, and in girls at 12. The older the person, the stiffer and more calcified the cartilage. Did you know that you can hear without the external ear? All the hearing apparatus is built inside the ear canal, but the external ear helps you localise where noise is coming from. For example, if you have no external ear and you are in a dark room and hear a noise, you won't know where the sound is coming from.

### *At what age can you have otoplasty?*

When deciding on the age and type of otoplasty to have done, the surgeon will consider the patient's maturity, appropriate ear development, evolving cartilage pliability, and the psychosocial stress from the deformity. For example, by three years of age, 90% of eventual ear growth is achieved; However, at six years, ear cartilage begins to harden significantly. After prominent ear correction in patients younger than six, studies by Mustarde found a 1.8% recurrence rate 10 years after the procedure. However, patients older than six at the time of surgery experienced a 30% increase in relapse rate.

Otoplasty can be performed on children of any age, but there are two age brackets that plastic surgeons recommend: one is before they start school and socialising to avoid potential bullying, and the other is when the child requests surgery. Older children are mature enough to become active participants in the decision-making process, and therefore post-operative care is optimal. This usually happens when they are in their early teens.

In newborns, doctors can use splints to help remould the ear cartilage to a more desirable shape and position, but this needs to be done in the first two weeks of life when it is believed that the circulating maternal hormones make the ear cartilage soft and pliable, and amenable to non-surgical change. However, after this time frame, remoulding with splints doesn't work. From a practical sense, this is extremely difficult to implement in a newborn.

In infants and young children, ear surgery is a decision that should be discussed and agreed upon by both parents. My third daughter, for example, inherited my ears, which are slightly protruding, but not bad enough to warrant surgery. I mentioned to my wife at my daughter's birth that we might consider splints to push her ears back. This was not well received, and the topic has never been raised again.

### *The consultation*

When consulting with a patient and their parents, I discuss the details of ear surgery, and the results they would like. I examine the shape, size, and placement of both my patient's ears to determine what sort of changes may be possible, even if only one needs pinning or reshaping. I also take photos of the ears and face to help determine the proportions of the patient's facial features.

### *How is the otoplasty performed?*

Otoplasty is typically done under general anesthesia. In adults, where the cartilage is harder, the procedure must be carried out by removing or repositioning cartilage after making a small incision in the ear. Then the common anatomical anomalies listed earlier are addressed with an otoplasty, and depending on your anatomy and desired changes, surgery is customised accordingly. The incision is hidden behind the ear, and the excess cartilage that makes the ear protrude is hitched and pulled back towards the skull, and anchored to the fascia overlying the bone. If normal folds are missing from the ear, they can be recreated by shaping the cartilage with permanent sutures or scraping the cartilage to contour it. Sometimes a combination of techniques is needed to get the desired result.

### *What are the risks?*

There are few risks associated with ear surgery, but as with any invasive surgery, there's always a potential for complications. The rare but potential risks associated with ear surgery are:

- Scarring, though most scars will be small, white, and unnoticeable
- Alterations in the sensitivity of the skin on or around your ears
- Bleeding or infection
- Asymmetry in the positioning of your ears due to changes that occur after surgery.

It's important to have regular follow-up visits to your doctor to ensure you are on the right track to recovery.

### *Will there be scarring?*

The location of incisions depends largely on what changes are desired. However, the incisions are in inconspicuous locations, either in the back of the ear where it connects to the head, or within the inner folds of the ear.

### *Recovery*

It's normal for ears to swell and feel tender following the procedure. There may also be redness around the affected area, and patients may experience tingling in the outer ear, though this will diminish over time. There is usually a heavy bandage around the head that we call a turban dressing, which stays on as long as practical. Once it is removed, I like to get my patients into a ski style headband to help protect the ears, especially when sleeping. For the first week of recovery, it's important that you rest, though you should still move around occasionally to keep blood flowing. To minimise discomfort, it's recommended that you recline, but keep your head elevated.

Approximately one week after the procedure, patients are reviewed in the clinic, and dressings changed. The stitches are usually self dissolving, and though recovery is different for each patient, you can resume light activity after one week. In two weeks, your final results will be visible, though small changes to the ears can occur for up to six months. I encourage all patients to sleep in the headband for the first month after surgery.

### *Samantha, 18, NSW

"I've been self-conscious about my large, protruding ears my whole life. I would try to cover them up with my hair. Sometimes I felt so insecure that I wouldn't want to leave the house. I still don't put my hair behind my ears out of habit. The kids at school would call me elephant ears, and if I missed something that was said, they'd say 'I can't believe you didn't hear us with those big ears.' Even one of my dad's friends told me 'You should probably get those fixed while you're still young.' I was horrified.

When I was 15, I watched a YouTube video about ear pinning; I saw the before and after pictures online, and the results looked really great! I went straight to my parents and asked if I could have this done. My mum had heard about Dr. Moradi's reputation and she suggested I see him for a consultation. My parents asked most of the basic questions. I was so excited about having this done, I wasn't nervous at all. I'd see other girls with small ears, and thought I was the only one with big ones. I just wanted to fit in and feel normal. I didn't want to feel like I was sticking out.

There's no prep necessary for otoplasty. I was asleep during the operation; I had never had anaesthesia before, so I felt weird when I woke up. I was in a lot of pain after surgery, and I took Tylenol, which helped a bit. The pain went away after about a week. My head was wrapped up with bandages, and I couldn't sleep on my side during recovery. I also had to be careful washing my hair. I used baby shampoo and my hair looked awful, but I was on a six-week holiday from school over Christmas so I didn't have to see anyone.

All my friends knew I was getting it done. It took a while before my ears looked natural, because they were kind of flat against my head in the beginning. My friends thought that they looked good. All I know is that I felt great! I think about it every day, and I can't even imagine having big ears again. I'm still an insecure person about my appearance, and there are other things I'd like to fix about myself, but I feel like if I keep having surgery I won't stop.

I've had a boyfriend for two years now, who is really supportive. He tells me that I look good the way I am. If you are a young girl with big ears or a big nose that you don't like, and you can afford to get them fixed – do it. Just know that you are still going to nitpick about other things you don't like about your appearance. Getting plastic surgery isn't going to change you as a person. If you're like me, you will always be self-critical. You can change things on the outside, but surgery won't solve all your problems and insecurities."

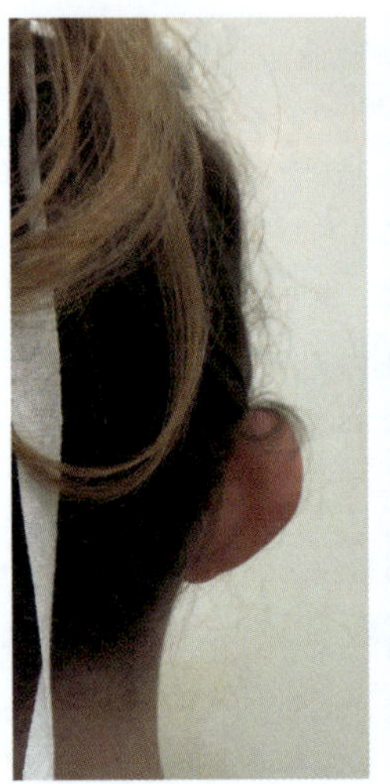
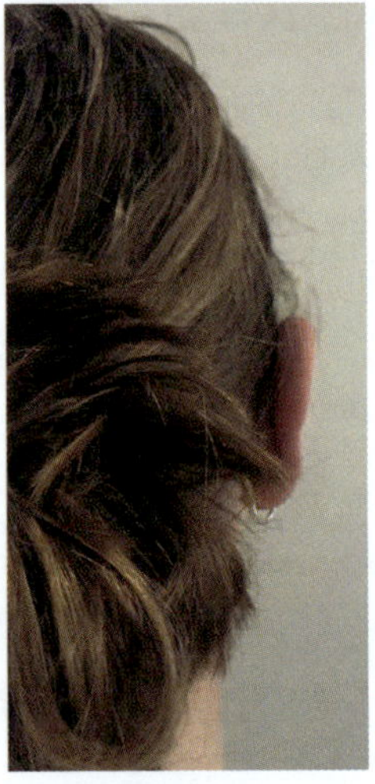

*Before and after otoplasty*

CHAPTER FIVE

# PARTS DOWN UNDER

It may not surprise you to learn that some women are self-conscious about the way their vaginas look. Because female genitalia are hidden, many wonder whether or not they are normal, and when young women see images of idealised and retouched female genitalia online, it creates anxiety about how they compare. The reasons women seek labiaplasty have been steeped in controversy in recent years, although several studies have found that patients with functional and appearance-related symptoms associated with long labia minora have high levels of satisfaction after the surgery and low complication rates. Many physicians have historically opposed the procedure, claiming that women with normal anatomy are unduly influenced by Brazilian waxing, online images, pornography, and promotion of designer vaginas to socially vulnerable women.

The influence of media images on women's interest in labiaplasty has also been the subject of several studies. In a 2016 article published in the *Aesthetic Surgery Journal*, scientist Gemma Sharp wrote that women who had undergone the procedure had seen more images of the female genitalia in the media and internalised their idealised form compared with women who had not undergone labiaplasty. In another article published in the same journal two years earlier, researchers Otto Placik and John Arkins discovered an increase in labiaplasty with a shift in *Playboy* magazine's focus from the breasts to the female genitalia.

Although other researchers have found that pornography influences women to have labiaplasty, there is little evidence to confirm that it has a major impact. In a 2011 study of 33 women seeking labiaplasty, Dr. Naomi Crouch, chair of the British Society of Paediatric and Adolescent Gynaecology, and colleagues, found that only 12% of those patients reported even viewing pornography, much less being influenced by it. Rather than agreeing that women are manipulated by the media, I believe that women who are unhappy with the appearance of their genitalia may turn to the internet to find out how to address their concerns, because it is the most accessible source of information. Common symptoms that patients complain about are:

- Physical symptoms
  - Tugging during intercourse
  - Discomfort wearing tight clothing
  - Uncomfortable twisting of labia
  - Visible labia in exercise clothing
  - Pain during intercourse
  - Exposure in a bathing suit.
- Psychological symptoms
  - Self-consciousness about appearance
  - Negative self-esteem
  - Less attractive to partner
  - Restrictive clothing choices
  - Negative impact on intimacy.

Women's bodies are incredibly diverse, and there's beauty in that diversity. Let's begin with an anatomy lesson.

## GENITAL ANATOMY

People often confuse the vagina and vulva. The vulva is the outside of the female genitalia that helps protect the sexual organs, vagina, and urinary opening from infection. The external genitalia has many parts, including the labia majora, labia minora, clitoris, and vestibule. The vagina, which is inside the body, performs several functions, including childbirth, as a passageway for menstrual blood, and for sexual intercourse.

## INNIES AND OUTIES

The terms innie and outie vagina can be misleading, as they refer to the external genitalia or the vulva. When people talk about innies or outies, they are typically referring to the labia majora and labia minora. These parts of the vulva are also called the lips. The labia majora are the larger outer lips,

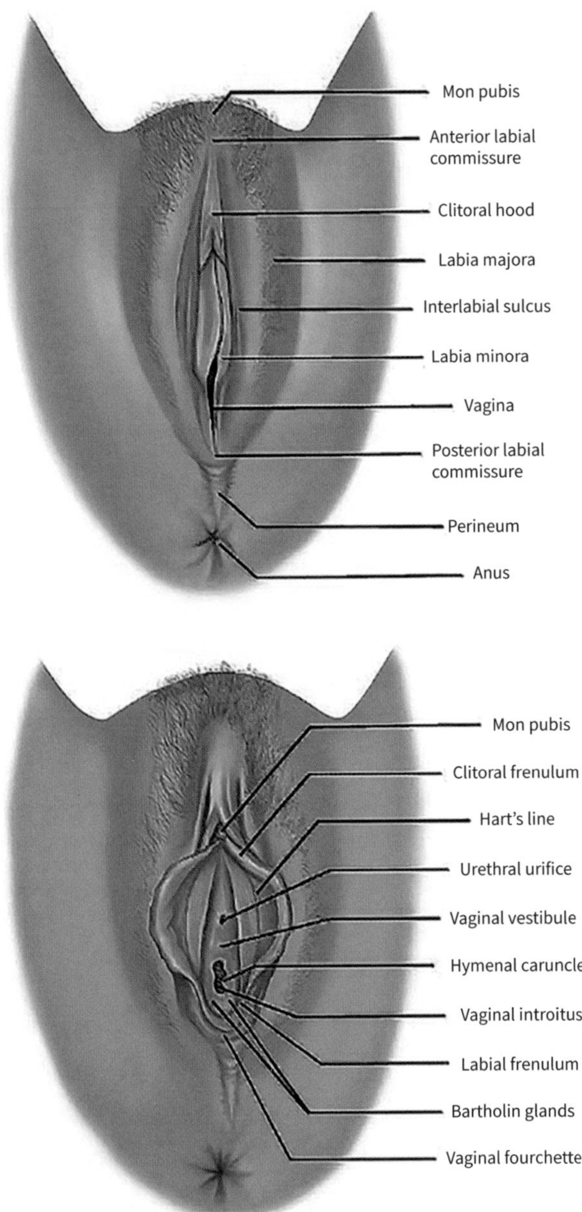
Mon pubis
Anterior labial commissure
Clitoral hood
Labia majora
Interlabial sulcus
Labia minora
Vagina
Posterior labial commissure
Perineum
Anus
Mon pubis
Clitoral frenulum
Hart's line
Urethral urifice
Vaginal vestibule
Hymenal caruncle
Vaginal introitus
Labial frenulum
Bartholin glands
Vaginal fourchette

and the labia minora are the smaller inner lips. Both types are anatomically normal and should not be a cause for concern. All external genitalia have a slightly different appearance – in other words, no two vulvas are the same.

According to one 2017 study, 56% of vulvas have visible labia minora or outies, which means that more than half of all women have labia minora that are longer than their labia majora. A more accurate name for this would be outie vulva. The size of the labia minora varies, and the fact is, some women have innies and others have outies – both are normal. When a patient sees a surgeon for a labiaplasty, she almost always wants to reduce the projection of the labia minora so that it doesn't protrude further than the labia majora, both standing and lying on their back.

## LABIA SYMMETRY

I discussed breast and face symmetry in previous chapters, and here's the deal about parts down under. Symmetry is rare in female genitalia. Just like many women have one breast that's larger than the other, the same is true for labia. The human body is not symmetrical; our hands are different sizes, and each half of our faces is slightly different too. Most labias are not symmetrical. Some are more symmetrical than others, but they are all normal and healthy.

## LABIA COLOUR

Some women have pink labia, and others are brown, reddish or purplish. Sometimes the labia are the same colour as the woman's skin, but often they are lighter or darker, just like the lips on your face. Variation in the colour of your labia is normal.

## LABIAPLASTY

This term has come to be associated with labia minora reduction, although any aesthetic intervention on the labia minora or majora could be called a labiaplasty. Labia minora reduction is the most commonly performed procedure. I've had patients come to me because they are embarrassed by a bulge under their clothing, or they feel uncomfortable when they're with a sexual partner. For some of these women labiaplasty can help. According to a 2016 survey by ASPS, the number of labiaplasty procedures has increased worldwide over the last few years by 45%.

### *What happens during surgery?*

A surgeon performing a labiaplasty will remove excess tissue to allow the lips of the labia minora to be tucked within the labia majora – the outer lips of the vulva. It is a simple procedure that can be done with general anaesthesia as a day surgical procedure. There are many techniques described, but common to all is the goal of reshaping and reducing the labia minora so it does not protrude further than the labia majora. The satisfaction rate of this surgery is very high, both in my practice and in studies that show a more than 90% satisfaction rate with complication rates of less than 5%.

### *Recovery*

For most women, recovery is quick and uncomplicated. Pain medication is recommended for a few days afterwards. Patients may want to take a week off from work to relax and heal, and wear loose clothes and a mini-pad for any minor bleeding. Most patients can resume normal activities within a month.

## MENSTRUATION

There was a time, not so long ago, when girls weren't taught about puberty and periods – and sadly some still remain in the dark. It was not uncommon for a girl to one day find herself covered in blood from her first period, terrified that she was bleeding to death. Menacing euphemisms such as the curse reflect attitudes about this biological benchmark. Thankfully, times have changed, as author Genevieve Kingston, whose mother died before she reached puberty, writes in her moving essay for *The New York Times*:

> *"When I was 3, my mother learned she had advanced breast cancer and immediately began assembling two gift boxes: one for my brother and one for me. Inside, she packed presents and letters for the milestones of our lives she would miss....When I got my first period and couldn't bring myself to talk to my father about it, a four-page letter (marked 'First Period') laid out practical advice: 'Take time to learn what interests you, what your opinions and feelings are, find your own sense of the world and which values you hold most dear.' As I read, I wanted to fall through the white, lightly textured page and into her arms. 'Please try not to lose yourself,' it continued. 'These are challenging years.'"*

This reminded me of my own letter to my daughters, and my wish to provide them with information and a bit of parental wisdom. With this goal in mind, I offer the following:

From the time of your first period (menarche) until it stops (menopause), the sole purpose of your monthly cycle is reproduction. If a fertilised egg does not implant in the wall of the uterus after ovulation, the lining sheds. This is your menstrual period. The average age of beginning menstruation is 12 and it ends at about 52. Menstruation happens about every 28 days – about 14 days after regular ovulation when there is no pregnancy. If the body does not ovulate, menstruation will be irregular.

Many hormonal changes occur before and during a period. It happens every month and it's the driving force behind your menstrual cycle. Believe it or not, the main players in this monthly process are in the brain – the hypothalamus and the pituitary gland – along with the ovaries. Technically, they work together to form the hypothalamic-pituitary-gonadal axis. When all goes well, ovulation, if no egg is fertilised, and menstruation will happen at regular intervals.

### *Monthly mood swings*

As hormone levels rise and fall during the menstrual cycle, they can affect the way you feel both physically and emotionally. This is known as premenstrual syndrome (PMS) and makes some women feel tired or irritable. Luckily, there are ways to ease PMS symptoms, such as eating lots of fresh fruit and vegetables, cutting back on processed and junk foods, and reducing salt and caffeine intake.

### *Follicular phase*

As your period begins and the built-up lining from the previous cycle is shed, your brain produces hormones that stimulate the ovaries to release estrogen and prepare an egg for ovulation. This is called the follicular phase. As estrogen levels rise, the lining of the uterus, or endometrium, begins to thicken or proliferate.

### *Ovulation phase*

In response to another change in hormone levels from your brain, the ovary releases an egg (oocyte) and ovulation occurs. This usually happens on day 14 of your cycle.

### *Luteal phase*

The follicle that releases the egg begins to shrink, and becomes a structure known as the corpus luteum. It continues to produce estrogen, but now begins to produce progesterone as well. Although both estrogen and progesterone are produced during this part of the cycle, concentrations of the latter dominate.

With the increase in progesterone, the lining of the uterus prepares for pregnancy. In the last half of the cycle, the uterine lining becomes thicker and more complex, with glands, blood vessels, and tissue swelling. These are all changes that prepare it for the process of implantation and pregnancy.

If implantation of a fertilised egg does not occur, the corpus luteum in the ovary continues to shrink, and estrogen and progesterone levels continue to fall. When this happens, the blood vessels that expand in the thickened lining constrict and cut off blood flow. The thickened lining, now without blood flow to support it, dies and is shed from the uterus.

## CHANGES IN PERIODS

Each woman's menstrual cycle is unique. Depending on the month, your period may come a few days early or late, and the menstrual flow may be heavy or light. Many factors can influence the hormone changes in your body, including:

- Stress
- Exercise
- Weight gain/loss
- Travel
- Illness.

Some women's cycles are more sensitive to fluctuations in hormone levels than others, and although it is normal for menstruation to vary, it is also normal for it to stay completely regular.

## MISSED PERIODS

Several factors can result in a late or missed period, such as stress, birth control, low body weight, or obesity. Some of these causes are harder to recognise than others, so it's important to consult a doctor if the cause is unclear.

It is not unusual to miss a period occasionally. If you're sexually active, however, the most common cause is pregnancy. Consider taking a pregnancy test if you are more than seven days late or have missed a period. If you are not pregnant, a missed period usually means that ovulation did not occur. The same things that can influence menstrual flow, like stress and exercise, can influence ovulation. As long as you have determined that you are not pregnant, it's okay to wait another month to see if your period comes. If you miss your period for two or three months in a row, talk to your doctor.

## PERIOD MYTHS AND MISCONCEPTIONS

Misconceptions about periods have been passed down for generations. Aside from being blatantly false, these superstitions contribute to gender-based taboos and discrimination. They can also make it harder for women to talk about their period – which leads to silence, shame, and misconceptions. Here are just a few of the age-old menstruation myths from around the world:

- Periods make you clumsy
- Tampons will break your hymen and make you impure
- Don't swim or take a bath during your period
- Camping is dangerous because the bears can smell period blood from far away
- If you touch any vegetable before or while pickling them, they won't pickle and will go bad
- You shouldn't visit anyone during your period
- If you slap a girl when she starts her first period, she will have beautiful rosy cheeks for the rest of her life
- If you shower with hot water when you have your period it will be a heavy flow
- Cold beverages will give you cramps
- If a woman touches flowers during her period, they will die
- Don't bake while menstruating, because the dough won't rise
- You can't get pregnant during your period
- Women's periods make them too emotional to be political leaders.

## PERIOD STRESS

A 2019 survey by Plan International UK found that more than half of girls aged 14–21 have missed school because they are embarrassed or worried about having their period. Nearly six in 10 (57%) say they have experienced negative comments – being told periods were dirty or disgusting, being mocked for their perceived mood or behaviour while menstruating, or being teased about leaking and sanitary products.

**What parents can do**

The earlier you begin talking to your daughter about what to expect when she gets her first period, the better. Plan on a series of conversations, not just one big reveal. If your child asks questions about menstruation, answer them openly and honestly. If she isn't asking questions, it's up to you to start the discussion before she reaches puberty.

You might begin by asking what she already knows. Clarify any misinformation, ask if your child has questions, and explain the basics. Mothers may want to share their experiences. Don't assume that your daughters will learn it all in school. Your child needs to know the facts about the menstrual cycle and all the changes that puberty brings. Friends often provide inaccurate information.

Talking to your daughter can help ease unfounded fears or anxiety, as well as positively influence her body image. Also, conversations about menstruation can lay the groundwork for future talks about dating and sexuality.

## THE PERIOD POSITIVE MOVEMENT

Here's what Terese Lann Welin of My Period is Awesome had to say about the stigma surrounding menstruation.

"Menstruation has, for as long as I can remember, been surrounded by shame and taboos. Growing up, no one told me that menstruation was shameful or dirty; I was just affected by societal norms to keep it hidden. In my whole life, I've perceived menstruation as something that is solely bad. It hurts, it's annoying, it makes me moody, and gives me breakouts. As a teenager, I talked about my period with close friends sometimes, but it was always in a bad way. What good is there even to say? I guess we all would just like to skip the days of bleeding if we could. Today, I work for the organisation My Period Is Awesome. Telling people that name always gives them a weird look on their faces: 'Periods, awesome? Huh, not mine!'

That is probably what I was thinking the first time I got in contact with MPIA, too. It's a good name because it sparks an interest and starts a conversation. When I was in university and about 24, I started studying periods and their connection to global health and human rights. At this stage of my life, I had been menstruating for 12 years. There was so much relatability to what I read on the current research. The menstrual stigma exists worldwide, and experiences I read from people across the planet happened to me in Sweden. Present evidence clearly shows that people do not feel comfortable talking openly about menstruation anywhere in the world. Society, through negative messages about menstrual cycles and negative answers to any mention of the menses, socially constructs menstruation as unfavourable.

Studies show that we only talk about our menstruation in negative terms because of the stigma attached to it. One researcher, M. McHugh, introduced the term 'menstrual moaning', which refers to people's negative communication about menstruation. McHugh emphasises that breaking the taboos by adopting a more positive and open language is a form of resistance. This resistance, talking openly about menstruation and breaking the secrecy, would then make people more resilient to menstrual shame.

The fact that we reiterate negative constructions about bleeding bodies as dirty, flawed, diseased, and deficient has an impact on our attitudes towards our bodies – which in turn perpetuates menstrual shame. McHugh mentions that positive conversations about menstruation are infrequent. Talking about menstrual experiences may be viewed as a form of activism: breaking the taboo and resisting the patriarchal norm. Scholars and activists show that we need to challenge, upset, and reverse the silence and shame concerning menstruation.

My period for sure isn't awesome. But the fact that I have a menstrual cycle is. Even though it hurts like hell, even though it is very annoying and expensive, I can say that my period is awesome. My internalised shame is deeply rooted. Writing this, I am 28 years old, and I've been reading menstruation research and working with period positive projects for several years, and I STILL experience shame. I've learned that it is a process, and awareness and openness are critical. It is okay to moan, and it is okay to talk openly about everything concerning your cycle."

You can follow Terese and My Period Is Awesome at #noperiodshame

## MENOPAUSE

The word menopause comes from the Greek words for month and cessation, referring to the final menstrual period. In reality, menopause, sometimes called the change, is a transition akin to puberty, where hormonal changes lead from one biological phase of life to another. Like menstruation, menopause is caused by changes in both the ovaries and the brain.

Women are born with a finite number of eggs, or oocytes. Over time, the supply and quality of oocytes decrease, affecting the production of estrogen and progesterone as well as the brain's response to these hormones. Medically, this time is known as the menopause transition. These hormonal changes often begin when a woman is in her mid-40s, and can last for years, typically producing symptoms such as menstrual irregularities, hot flushes, vaginal dryness, depression, difficulty sleeping, and brain fog. Here are the stages:

- *Pre-menopause.* The body has not begun menopause
- *Perimenopause.* The body slowly begins to reduce its estrogen production. This can occur in one year or gradually over several years. Menopause symptoms may start to occur at the tail end of this stage. Periods continue, and a woman can still become pregnant
- *Menopause.* The body stops producing estrogen, and there is no menstrual cycle for 12 consecutive months
- *Post-menopause.* The years following menopause.

Eventually, a woman will have her last menstrual period – an event that typically occurs when she is about 51. Hormonal changes during this time can increase women's risk of conditions such as heart disease, stroke, dementia and osteoporosis. On the plus side, women may also be relieved by the end of menstrual cramps and heavy or irregular periods, or the risk of an unexpected pregnancy.

Because many women are unaware of the basic biology of menopause, they don't know what to expect when they no longer have a regular period. Menopause isn't a sentence of biological irrelevance. Women should dispel the notion that their worth is tied to age and reproductive capacity. Instead, they should embrace this new phase of life.

## MENOPAUSE MISCONCEPTIONS

Here are a few common falsehoods about menopause:

- *You can't get pregnant during menopause.* You can get pregnant during the process of menopause or perimenopause when your cycle may be irregular. After one full year without a period, when you are considered through menopause, you can no longer become pregnant, although you may still be at risk for sexually transmitted diseases (STDs).

- *Every woman gets hot flushes.* Each woman has a different menopause experience. Some have hot flushes. Some have insomnia. Some don't experience any symptoms.
- *All menopausal women get fat.* Although many women do gain weight during perimenopause and beyond, it is not inevitable. As we age, our energy requirements lessen and our metabolism slows down, making weight loss more difficult. Combine this with a sedentary lifestyle and unhealthy diet, and middle-aged women will be fighting a bulging middle. Nevertheless, exercise, proper nutrition, and a reasonably portioned whole-food, plant-based diet can help keep you fit and trim throughout your lifetime.

**Resources**

- Puberty for Girls/Health Direct, www.healthdirect.gov.au
- Parenting Website, Raising Children, www.raisingchildren.net.au
- The Australasian Menopause Society, www.menapause.org.au
- Menopause Support Group, Join Facebook community with over 11,000 members from 80 countries worldwide.

## CHAPTER SIX

# BORN THIS WAY

I remember my joy when I learned that I was going to be a father for the first time. I felt some nervous anticipation, too. As a plastic surgeon who works at the Sydney Childrens' Hospital, I knew about all the things that could go wrong prenatally, so my elation was tempered with worry about possible complications. I felt the same twinge of anxiety – and delight – with all three of my daughters. Like most parents, I silently counted their fingers and toes after each birth, and breathed a sigh of relief as I held our newborns and gazed into their perfect little faces.

Unfortunately, this is not the case for all parents. About 3–4% of babies are born with some type of birth defect. A birth defect is a health problem or a physical abnormality that can be mild or severe. They can be inherited or caused by something in the environment, and in many cases, the cause is unknown. These abnormalities often require medical or surgical care, and having a child who is born different from the norm can take an emotional toll on families. This chapter is not about the more serious congenital abnormalities, but rather the common conditions we see at Sydney Children's Hospital that can be treated with surgery or some kind of medical intervention.

## CLEFT LIP AND CLEFT PALATE

Cleft lips and cleft palates are amongst the most common birth anomalies affecting children worldwide. This incomplete formation of the upper lip or roof of the mouth can occur individually, or both defects may occur together. The conditions can vary in severity, and may involve one or both sides of the mouth. Surgery is required to repair both.

### *What causes a cleft lip?*

As a baby develops during pregnancy, body tissue and special cells from each side of the head grow toward the centre of the face and join together to make the face. The joining of tissue forms the lips and mouth, and a cleft lip occurs if the tissue that makes up the lip does not come together completely before birth. This results in an opening in the upper lip, which can be a small slit or it can be a large opening that goes through the lip into the nose. A cleft lip can be on one or both sides of the lip, or in the middle of the lip, which occurs very rarely. Children with a cleft lip can also have a cleft palate. Approximately eight out of every 10,000 babies are born with a cleft lip.

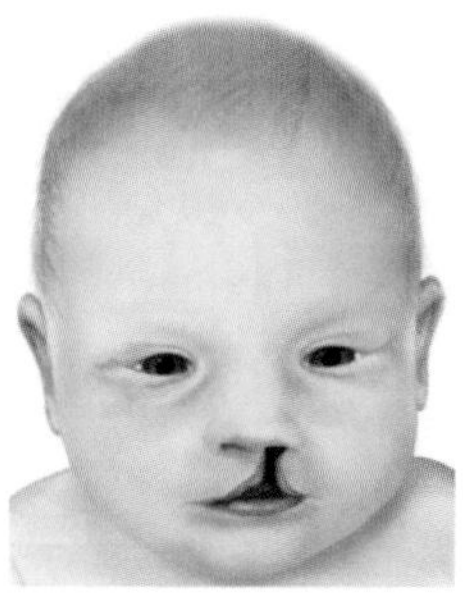

*Cleft lip*

### *What is a cleft palate?*

The roof of the mouth is formed between the sixth and ninth weeks of pregnancy, and a cleft palate occurs when the tissue from the palate does not join together completely. For some babies, both the front and back parts of the palate are open, while for others, only part of the palate is open.

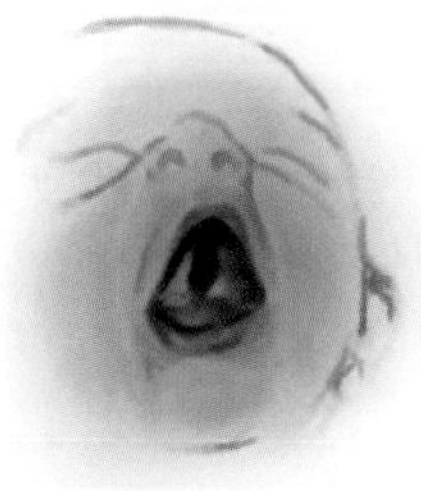

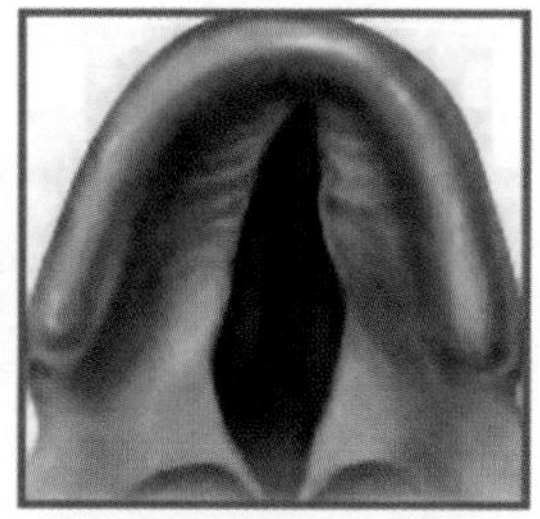

*Cleft palate*

### *Other problems*

The medical term for these birth defects is orofacial clefts. Children born with a cleft lip (with or without a cleft palate) or a cleft palate alone often have problems with feeding and speaking clearly, and are susceptible to ear infections. They may also develop hearing and dental problems.

### *It takes a team*

Early intervention by a team of specialists is often called on to evaluate and manage treatments for a cleft lip and/or cleft palate. Treatment can include surgical repair of the cleft, feeding recommendations, speech rehabilitation, and dental restoration. The specialists may include a:

- Plastic surgeon
- Paediatrician
- Paediatric dentist
- Orthodontist
- Otolaryngologist
- Lactation specialist
- Occupational therapist
- Auditory or hearing specialist
- Speech-language pathologist
- Genetic counsellor
- Psychologist
- Social worker.

At the earliest stages, feeding, growth, and development will be the most important priorities for your baby's cleft-related care. Often with a cleft palate, the infant will not be able to breastfeed due to problems creating oral suction. If this is the case, specialised bottles or feeding tubes may be necessary to help them get enough to eat.

### *Surgery for a cleft lip*

Surgery to repair a cleft lip is highly individualised. The procedure is intended to close the cleft defect, and also to help the child function.

Cleft lip repair, which involves reconstruction of the lip to create a more normal appearance, includes:

- Closure of the cleft resulting in a scar located within or near the typical features of the upper lip
- Formation of a cupid's bow curve along the center of the upper lip
- Establishing adequate distance between the upper lip and nose
- Reattaching the separated muscles of the mouth, allowing for the lip and mouth to function normally.

Clefts of the upper lip typically affect the shape of the nose and additional procedures may be needed to:

- Restore nasal symmetry and nostril shape
- Straighten and create adequate length for the columella tissue that separates the nostrils.

### *Surgery for a cleft palate*

Because the palate creates the floor of the nasal cavity, it is responsible for facilitating normal speech. As such, surgery to repair a cleft palate includes:

- Separating the mouth and nasal tissues by closing the defect
- Re-establishing soft palate muscle function to promote normal speech
- Recreating normal relation of the soft palate to the auditory canal and Eustachian or auditory tube, which links the nasopharynx to the middle ear, to allow for normal hearing
- Promoting the normal growth and development of the upper jaw and teeth
- Repairing, when appropriate, defects in the gumline to allow for permanent tooth growth.

Treatments for children with orofacial clefts vary, depending on the severity of the cleft and the child's age and needs. Surgery to repair a cleft lip usually occurs in the first few months of life, and is recommended within the first

12 months. Surgery to repair a cleft palate is recommended within the first 18 months of life, or earlier if possible. Many children will need additional surgical procedures as they get older. Surgery can improve the look and appearance of a child's face, as well as improve breathing, hearing, and speech and language development. Children born with orofacial clefts may also need special dental or orthodontic care, or speech therapy.

The good news is that, with treatment, most children with orofacial clefts do well and lead a healthy life, although some may have issues with self-esteem if they are concerned about looking different.

### *Causes and risk factors*

The causes of orofacial clefts are unknown, and are thought to be a combination of genes and other factors, such as what the mother comes in contact with in her environment, what she eats or drinks, or certain medications taken during pregnancy. A cleft lip and palate may also be part of a random or genetically determined syndrome.

Here are some of the possible causes and risk factors according to the latest research studies:

- *Smoking.* Women who smoke during pregnancy are more likely to have a baby with an orofacial cleft than women who do not smoke
- *Diabetes.* Women with diabetes diagnosed before pregnancy have an increased risk of having a child with a cleft lip with or without a cleft palate
- *Use of certain medicines.* Women who have used certain medicines to treat epilepsy, such as topiramate or valproic acid, during the first three months of pregnancy, have an increased risk of having a baby with cleft lip with or without a cleft palate.

More research on cleft lips and cleft palates, and how to prevent them continues to be done.

*Diagnosis*

Orofacial clefts, especially a cleft lip with or without a cleft palate, can be diagnosed during pregnancy by a routine ultrasound. They can also be diagnosed after the baby is born, especially a cleft palate. However, sometimes certain types of cleft palates, such as a submucous cleft palate or bifid uvula may not be discovered until later in life.

## MICHELLE AND CADE

Michelle and her son Cade, who was born with a cleft lip and palate, shared their story with the Centers for Disease Control and Prevention (CDC). Both mother and son relied on their faith for support, and Cade did not let his disability define him as a person.

**Michelle's story**

*"He has learned to define his disability, not let it define him."*

"My son Cade was born in April of 2000 with a severe case of cleft lip and palate. I didn't learn about Cade's cleft during my pregnancy. After his birth, I had a lot to absorb and learn very quickly. Even though we were devastated and scared at first, my husband and I immediately embraced the challenges we knew we faced, and we were just as proud of our new son as if he had been born without a birth defect. We knew that God had given Cade to us for a reason, and we spent the first few months of Cade's life educating ourselves about his condition and things we could do to make Cade's life as normal as possible. Although there were things we had to do differently, we tried very hard to treat Cade as though there was nothing different about him. Before his first corrective surgery, we proudly showed him off, took pictures of him, and sent him to daycare as though there was nothing different about him. We focused on educating everyone we came in contact with, rather than sheltering him at home.

When Cade began school, sometimes the other children would tease him. As much as it broke my heart when he was bullied, we explained that everyone gets made fun of and that we all have insecurities. We asked our family and close friends to share their own experiences and insecurities, and encouraged Cade to address his differences. When he was the star of the week in school, he would bring in pictures from infancy and educate his classmates and teachers about his condition. Before each surgery, I would join him at school to talk about the surgery in front of his class. As a result, the other children became supportive and protective of Cade rather than teasing him once they knew more about what he was going through.

Cade has had five reconstructive surgeries, five sets of ear tubes, and has many more surgeries to come. I admire Cade for his determination, confidence, and his caring and outgoing personality. He has learned to define his disability, not let it define him, and to use it to help others by telling his story."

**Cade's story**

"God has made me this way for a reason, and I feel His reason was for me to help show other kids and adults that it's okay to have a disability. It shouldn't hold you back. It has never stopped me from doing anything. Sure there are things I don't like about myself, but overall I am happy with the way I look. My goals are to continue to make people feel better about themselves, and strive to become a professional baseball player. If I had a message it would be to say 'Look at me, not my disability!' You have a gift not a disability, so hold your head high and go for your dreams."

## BIRTHMARKS

A birthmark is a coloured mark on or under the skin that's present at birth or develops shortly afterwards. They are extremely common, and in fact it's estimated that more than 10% of babies have a birthmark. Some fade with time, whilst others become more pronounced. Birthmarks may be caused by extra pigment-producing cells in the skin, or by blood vessels that do not grow normally. Most are painless and harmless, but in rare cases they can cause complications or are associated with other conditions, so it's a good idea to get all birthmarks checked.

## TYPES OF BIRTHMARKS

Most birthmarks will fit into one of the following two categories:

1. *Vascular birthmarks.* These are associated with blood vessels under the skin, and are typically red or pink
2. *Pigmented birthmarks.* These occur due to pigment changes within the skin, and can be brown, black, or bluish.

## VASCULAR BIRTHMARKS

Vascular anomalies fall into three unique groups – haemangiomas, vascular, and lymphatic malformations – based on the endothelial characteristics or lining of the blood vessels.

## HAEMANGIOMAS

Haemangiomas are a collection of small immature blood vessels, sometimes called strawberry marks because the surface of some looks a bit like a strawberry. Haemangiomas can be superficial or deep in the skin or a combination of the two, seen as a raised red area on the surface of the skin, and as a bluish swelling of abnormal blood vessels deeper in the skin. Occasionally haemangiomas may occur internally.

Haemangiomas have a defined natural history characterised by distinct periods of proliferation; in other words, there is a growth phase, plateau or rest phase, and involution or shrinkage phase. They are not present at birth, but become apparent within a few days or weeks, and grow rapidly in the first three to six months, increasing in size and sometimes in redness. As a general rule, 50% disappear by the age of five, 60% by six, and 70% by the age of seven.

Because of the natural tendency of haemangiomas to shrink over time, the treatment has largely been a watch and wait approach. Surgical intervention has only been needed for lesions in cosmetically sensitive areas such as the eyelid and nose, or functionally significant areas such as around the airway. In the past, the treatment has been surgical, but a serendipitous finding a number of years ago has greatly changed the management approach to hemangiomas. A heart medication called propanolol was being used on a child with heart failure who also had a haemangioma in the trachea. Doctors treating the child noticed that after being given the medication, the haemangioma started to shrink and involute much faster than expected.

## WHAT IS PROPRANOLOL?

Propranolol is a beta-blocker class of medications, used to slow the rhythm of the heart. Some nerves release a chemical called noradrenaline when they are stimulated, which in turn stimulates beta adrenergic receptors. These can cause a variety of effects. For instance, if the beta adrenergic receptors in the heart are stimulated, the heart pumps harder and faster than before, so more blood is pumped around the body. Beta-blocker medicines block the beta adrenergic receptors and stop them being stimulated, therefore slowing the heart rate.

Whilst it is still unclear how propanolol helps with haemagiomas, one theory is that by blocking the beta adrenergic receptors, propranolol can make blood vessels narrower, which decreases the amount of blood flowing through them, which reduces the colour and makes them softer. Growth of the haemangioma cells is also limited by propranolol so that the haemangioma starts to shrink. The beneficial effects are usually seen quickly.

## VASCULAR MALFORMATIONS

Vascular malformations, on the other hand, are present at birth but may not be clinically evident until early childhood. They result from morphologic errors in vascular development, and purportedly originate in utero, arising as early as the first trimester.

Unlike haemangiomas, vascular malformations grow commensurately with the child, and do not undergo spontaneous involution. Certain lesions may expand suddenly following trauma, sepsis, or hormonal changes. Vascular malformations can be further subclassified based on flow characteristics and/or the predominant diseased vessel. Two main categories exist: fast-flow lesions, such as arterial malformations, arteriovenous malformations, and arteriovenous fistulas, and slow-flow lesions, such as capillary malformations, lymphatic malformations, and venous malformations.

## CAPILLARY OR SALMON PATCH MALFORMATIONS

Salmon patches are nests of blood vessels that appear as small, pink, flat marks on the skin. These are known as macular stains, which show only dilated capillaries without additional pathologic findings on histologic examination, and fade between the neonatal period and the first two years of life. Salmon patches can appear on the back of the neck, where they are sometimes called a stork bite, between the eyes as an angel's kiss, or on the forehead, nose, upper lip, or eyelids. Some fade as the baby grows, but patches on the back of the neck usually don't go away. All salmon patches are noncancerous and require no treatment.

## PORT WINE STAIN

Port wine stains are vascular anomalies in the dermal layer of the skin. They begin as a flat, pinkish-red mark at birth, and gradually become darker and reddish-purple with age. Capillary malformations have been found to occur in three out of every 1,000 births and they have an equal male/female distribution, but are progressive, with a tendency to darken, thicken, and become more nodular with age. Capillary malformations can be located on the trunk, limbs, or face, and facial lesions can not only result in soft-tissue hypertrophy, i.e. the enlargement of an organ or tissue from the increase in size of its cells, but also have associated underlying skeletal and orbital changes that require earlier intervention or surgery. Former Soviet leader Mikhail Gorbachev famously sported a large port wine birthmark on his forehead.

Whilst port wine stains can be associated with several syndromes, they are usually isolated and benign. Treatment is very much tailored to both the cosmetic and functional restoration of normal anatomy, and includes laser therapy, specific medication such as steroids targeting cellular growth of the lesion, and surgery. Like cleft lip and palate surgery, treatment for port wine stains in children or young people is typically done at a multidisciplinary specialised clinic such as a children's hospital similar to the one I work at in Sydney.

## LYMPHATIC MALFORMATIONS

Lymphatic malformations are slow-flow anomalies of the lymphatic channels. They occur in both genders, and can be subclassified as macrocystic, microcystic, or mixed anomalies based on the size of the lymphatic channels. Macrocystic lesions have been observed to undergo spontaneous involution, whereas microcystic lesions do not involute spontaneously.

Clinically, lymphatic malformations occur most often in the neck region, followed by the axilla or armpit, trunk, and extremities. Fifty percent of these lesions are discovered at birth, and 90% are evident by age two, although some may not be found until early childhood or adolescence. Lymphatic malformations are often associated with skeletal and soft-tissue overgrowth. Facial lymphatic malformations can present with skeletal enlargement and distortion, malocclusion, and mandibular overgrowth. This is a progressive process, purportedly the result of lymphatic overgrowth within the inner canal of the bone causing it to grow too.

Facial lymphatic malformations can also cause enlarged soft tissue structures, such as the tongue and mouth. Extremity malformations produce gigantism associated with both bony and soft-tissue overgrowth. Lymphatic malformations are treated with nonsurgical and surgical methods or, more commonly, a combination of both. Sclerotherapy, a technique where an agent is injected into the lymphatic channels, damaging their inner lining, has surfaced as an accepted method for the treatment of macrocystic lymphatic malformations. Microcystic lesions do not respond well to sclerosant therapy, however elastic support garments and sequential compression devices can be used.

Surgery is usually a last resort for the treatment of lymphatic malformations where there are functional limitations, intolerable symptoms, and altered aesthetics. The goal of surgery is to completely cut out the lesion, because transected and incompletely excised lesions often recur. However, complete removal of the lesion is seldom possible, because the lymphatic malformation often involves normal anatomy that must be preserved, and surgery is routinely staged over months, with only specific anatomical areas addressed at any one time.

## VENOUS MALFORMATIONS

Venous malformations are the most prevalent vascular malformation, and are frequently found in the head and neck region. Although present at birth, they are occasionally not evident until later in life because of a very slow flow with gradual venous dilation. Venous malformations appear as compressible masses located under the skin with an associated deep blue discoloration on the exterior of the skin. Although they generally grow with the child, trauma and hormonal changes can cause rapid expansion of these often painful lesions – specifically in the morning as a result of blood not moving freely within the venous system. The slowing of the blood flow causes micro clots within the lesion that become painful, firm, calcified masses.

Treatment for venous malformations is directed to those lesions causing functional limitations, pain, or aesthetic deformity. Similar to lymphatic malformations, treatments include elastic compression garments, sclerosing agents, and surgery. Compression garments help with the reduction of swelling and pain in an affected limb, and, in addition, prophylactic aspirin can be administered daily to prevent painful thrombotic events and clot formation. Sclerosants constitute the first line of treatment for venous malformations, and surgery is a last resort, saved for those with severe symptoms or functional limitations such as bleeding, pain, and nerve compression, well-localised lesions that can easily be removed, and lesions causing aesthetic concerns for the patient.

## ARTERIOVENOUS MALFORMATION

An arteriovenous malformation (AVM) is an abnormal tangle of blood vessels connecting arteries and veins, which disrupts normal blood flow and oxygen circulation. Arteries are responsible for taking oxygen-rich blood from the heart to the brain, and veins carry the oxygen-depleted blood back to the lungs and heart. AVMs are typically recognised at birth, but often misdiagnosed as capillary malformations or haemangiomas. Below is the staging system physicians use to describe the progression of AVM lesions:

- Stage I: initially quiescent, presenting as warm pink-blue macules
- Stage II: proceed to expand, with pulsations, thrills, and bruits
- Stage III: subsequently become destructive, with pain, bleeding, or ulceration
- Stage IV: finally decompensate, resulting in congestive heart failure.

Periods of rapid growth are found after trauma, and at times when the body is under the influence of hormonal changes during puberty. Treatment for AVMs should be based on the clinical stage of the lesion on presentation. Smaller, well-localised Stage I lesions can reliably be excised and reconstructed as needed. Larger, more diffuse AVMs are best managed with superselective arterial embolisation, where the radiologist injects an ablative agent within or close to the damaged vessels, and these induce destruction and blockage of the lining of the blood vessels. This procedure shrinks the tumour by depriving it of the oxygen-carrying blood and other substances it needs to grow. It is followed by surgical resection and reconstruction 24 to 48 hours after the embolisation.

## PIGMENTED BIRTHMARKS OR CAFE-AU-LAIT SPOTS

A birthmark named for a beverage, cafe-au-lait spots are smooth and oval, and range in colour from light to medium brown. Café-au-lait macules are usually present at birth or appear in early infancy, and are typically found on the torso, buttocks, and legs. They sometimes become apparent later in infancy, especially after exposure to the sun, which darkens the colour, but are generally not considered a problem.

They may be isolated or associated with systemic diseases such as neurofibromatosis, where tumours grow in the nervous system, and other conditions such as McCune-Albright syndrome, a rare genetic disorder affecting the bone, skin and endocrine systems. The overall prevalence of café-au-lait macules varies with race:

- 0.3% of Caucasians
- 0.4% of Chinese
- 3% of Hispanics
- 18% of African Americans.

Isolated café-au-lait macules are invariably solitary and therefore benign. More than three in a Caucasian or more than five in an African American are uncommon, and should lead to systemic evaluation, referral, and close follow-up as they are invariably linked to a syndrome. The brown colour of a café-au-lait macule is due to a melanin pigment, which is produced in the skin by melanocyte cells in the outer layer of the skin, which are the cells that form melanomas later in life. The other cell type, keratinocytes, lead to the other two common skin cancers: squamous cell carcinoma (SCC) and basal cell carcinoma (BCC).

The following are important facts to know about café-au-lait spots:

- The epidermal melanocytes of an isolated café-au-lait macule have excessive numbers of melanosomes or intracellular pigment granules
- The café-au-lait macules associated with NF type 1 and other syndromes have increased proliferation of epidermal melanocytes
- A café-au-lait macule is not classified as a congenital melanocytic naevus.

No medical treatment is required to treat café-au-lait spots. Lasers can help fade the colour of the lesions, but they do invariably return. Surgical removal needs to be carefully planned and the risks and rewards discussed with the parents, the major issue being that you are exchanging a benign, natural-looking lesion for a scar or skin graft.

## CONGENITAL NAEVI OR MOLES

Congenital naevi are moles that appear at birth and occur in 1% of newborns. The surface may be flat, raised, or bumpy, and these moles can grow anywhere on the body. A melanocytic naevus is an abnormal collection of melanocytes in an ectopic location, so that instead of the melanocytes residing in the basal layer of the skin's epidermis, they are present in all layers of the skin, its appendages and surrounding tissue. Congenital melanocytic naevi are thought to develop between weeks five and 25 of gestation. Why they occur remains unknown, but one theory is there is an over-representation of hepatic growth factors that help regulate the proliferation of melanocytes in utero. The overexpression of hepatic growth factors results in excessive and abnormal accumulations of melanocytes in the skin, classified according to their projected adult surface diameter:

- Small is less than 1.5 cm in diameter
- Medium is 1.5 cm to 20 cm
- Large is more than 20 cm.

Classification has been modified to consider large congenital melanocytic naevi as 11 to 20 cm in diameter, and lesions larger than 20 cm are considered giant. This number translates to an estimated diameter of 9 cm on an infant's head or 6 cm on their body. The incidence of giant congenital melanocytic naevi is 1:20,000. Whilst most moles are not dangerous, there remains great controversy with respect to the risk of malignant transformation into a melanoma, the deadliest type of skin cancer.

Historically, it has been common practice to aim for complete excision of giant congenital melanocytic naevi, based on reports that there is high risk that up to 8–12% will turn into melanomas, and on the assumption that surgical excision may reduce this risk. Both claims remain controversial, and have been challenged by recent data. The over-reporting of the risk of melanoma had been exaggerated in past studies as a result of a reporting bias in small populations referred to specialised centres, and a less accurate study of the microscopic structure of tissues.

Fortunately, recent studies show the overall incidence of melanoma to be lower (0.7–2.9%) than once believed, although this rate is still higher than that in the general population (0.6%). Fifty percent of these malignancies arise in the first three years of life, 60% by childhood, and 70% by puberty. The risk of melanoma appears to be higher in lesions that are larger than 20 cm projected adult surface, have multiple satellite lesions near the primary lesion, and are located on the trunk.

In a questionnaire study of 349 congenital melanocytic naevi patients from the Great Ormond Street Hospital in London, 12% of all cases of melanoma and death occurred in patients with either giant (> 60 cm) or multiple naevi, the rate of melanoma being 14% in this group as opposed to an overall rate of 1.4% for all patients.

There has been a paradigm shift over the last decade with regards to the treatment of giant melanocytic naevi, the result of reduced malignant concerns in the literature along with the limitations of surgery in achieving acceptable aesthetic results. Hence weighing malignant risk against aesthetic outcome has become more challenging for the plastic surgeon, patient, and family.

## DOES SURGERY REDUCE THE RISK OF MELANOMA?

There is no evidence that surgical treatment reduces the risk of melanoma, although according to a 2014 study published by surgeons at the Hospital for Sick Children in Toronto, there are several valid arguments for this conclusion:

1. The number of melanoma cases in most reported cohorts is too small to allow proper risk analysis. Also, most study groups are not controlled for

surgery, and include mixed populations of patients who had undergone surgery and those patients who had not

2. Data suggesting lower rates of melanoma following surgery are incomplete with respect to original size of lesions and extent of excision. This may skew the results, because smaller versus larger lesions probably have higher rates of complete excision, but also inherently carry a lower risk of melanoma regardless of surgery, which may falsely suggest that complete excision reduces the risk of melanoma
3. The risk of melanoma may be a generic biological risk unrelated directly to the presence of a specific congenital melanocytic naevus. This is supported by findings that melanoma often arises elsewhere from the naevus, either in normal skin or in the central nervous system.

The three commonly agreed indications for surgery are:

1. The presence of high-risk features, namely size, trunk location, and irregular shape. If complete resection is impossible, at least partial excision of those parts of the lesion that are most troubling is indicated. We clinicians should refrain from complete excision in cases where reconstruction options cause "mutilated appearance or function"
2. Complaints of itchiness, rash, or foul-smelling discharge from the lesion. Partial excision may be performed with the goal of functional relief
3. Probably the most challenging factor in weighing the risks versus benefits of surgery in congenital melanocytic naevi patients is predicting the post-operative cosmetic benefits and quality-of-life outcomes for the individual patient.

## HOW ARE BIRTHMARKS REMOVED?

In most cases, surgery to remove a small birthmark can be done as an outpatient procedure, which means that doctors use local anaesthesia, and the child can return home on the same day. Frequently, surgery to remove small birthmarks can be done in less than an hour. Surgeons inject the anaesthetic into the surrounding skin to eliminate pain, and then use a small scalpel to remove the birthmark. The small incision is closed with stitches that dissolve on their own within a week. For larger birthmarks, or those deeper in the skin, surgeons can use a combination of techniques to minimise scarring and prevent disfigurement. For example, if a large mole is present on a child's cheek, surgery can be done in stages: during the first procedure, surgeons remove a section from the middle of the birthmark, and then wait several weeks for the incision to heal. This may be repeated two or three times before the final section of the birthmark, now much smaller in size, is removed, which reduces the size of the incision required for final removal, shrinking the length of the scar.

Another technique is called tissue expansion. In this procedure, surgeons implant a small balloon beneath healthy skin next to the birthmark. In the weeks before surgery to remove the birthmark, this balloon is slowly expanded, and new healthy skin cells grow over it to create an extra flap of skin. During surgery to remove the birthmark, surgeons use this new flap of skin to cover the area where the birthmark used to be, and the new skin heals with minimal scarring.

## BIRTHMARK MYTH

It was once believed that if a pregnant woman had a food craving she didn't satisfy that her child would be born with a beauty mark in the shape of that food.

CHAPTER SEVEN

# THE HUNGER GAMES

## (ANOREXIA AND OTHER EATING DISORDERS)

One of the most important messages I can convey to my daughters is that confidence comes from how you *feel* about your body, not from how you look. We all have a certain perception about our body image, and sometimes we have to work at feeling good about ourselves. It can be difficult to feel confident when messages from the media make us feel less so (See Chapter Eight, page 143, *Your Selfie Image*), and at times self-criticism is influenced by peers, coaches, or family.

For some, having a negative body image can cause an obsession with food, weight, or shape. Although eating disorders (ED) affect people of any gender at any age, they're most often found in teens and young women, and in fact studies show up to 13% of young people develop an eating disorder by the age of 20. Contrary to some beliefs, an ED is not a lifestyle choice or a cry for attention – it is a psychological condition. Severe cases can have serious health consequences, and may result in death if left untreated.

One great resource for eating disorders in Australia is the Butterfly Foundation, which reported a 13% increase in calls from adolescents including children as young as 10 during the pandemic. This was gut-wrenching for me to learn, as my eldest daughter is 10. In 2021, the federal budget allocated $13 million to build a National Eating Disorder Research Centre with another $8.25 million in additional funding for treatment. Clinician and helpline leader at the Foundation Amelia Trinick says "We're seeing more and more parents talking about their young ones changing their eating habits based on anxiety and things like bullying."

Journalist Madonna King, author of *Ten-ager. What Your Daughter Needs to Know About the Transition from Child to Teen*, said 10 is the new start of adolescence, and her research has confirmed eating disorders and self harm are emerging in younger children. "The most common two words from my research among 10-year-olds are "fitting in," King said. "They tend to be tolerant of their friends, but brutally judgemental about themselves."

## WHAT ARE EATING DISORDERS?

Over a million Australians currently have some kind of eating disorder. There are six main types of EDs, each involving extreme and unhealthy behaviours having to do with food, and they dovetail with BDD, in that there is often a perceived concern about body shape or weight. Here are the different types.

## ANOREXIA NERVOSA

Anorexia nervosa is a well-known eating disorder, which generally develops during adolescence and continues to adulthood. Anorexics view themselves as overweight, even if they are dangerously thin. They constantly weigh themselves, avoid eating certain types of food, and drastically restrict their calories. Common symptoms of anorexia nervosa include:

- Being dangerously underweight
- Extremely restricted eating patterns
- An intense fear of gaining weight and obsessive behaviours to avoid weight gain
- An unrelenting desire to be thin, and an unwillingness to maintain a healthy weight
- Self-esteem tied to body weight and shape
- A distorted body image and denial that they're seriously underweight.

Anorexia is also closely linked with OCD. For example, many anorexics are preoccupied with food. Some may obsessively collect recipes, hoard food, or binge-watch cooking shows. Many seek to control their environment, and find it difficult to be spontaneous or to eat in public. Some anorexics lose weight by dieting, fasting, and excessive exercise. Others will eat large quantities of food, and purge afterwards by vomiting or taking laxatives and diuretics. The damage that anorexia inflicts on one's health over time includes brittle hair and nails, thinning bones, and infertility. In severe cases, it can result in heart, brain, and organ failure, as well as death.

## *Alyse

*"I fantasised about a false ideal of beauty."*

"Somewhere along the way, I accepted the lie that I wasn't enough. A boyfriend I loved left me for someone else, and I felt like my life had no direction. These things weighed on me daily, and I told myself if I was smarter, I'd have this figured out. If I was prettier, he wouldn't have broken up with me. If I was thinner, I'd be prettier.

Amidst all the things I *couldn't* control, there was something I *could*: my weight. When I compared myself to women in magazines and movies, I wasn't enough. I fantasised about a false ideal of beauty. I'd stand in front of mirrors while grabbing at my thighs and waist, imagining how great it'd be if there was less. How pretty I'd be then. How maybe I'd finally be *enough*.

I'd skip meals and work out in the pursuit of some undefined goal weight; I'd simply know it when I saw it. I ran some, but only when I couldn't make it to the gym or wanted an extra little burst of cardio. My body was something I could control, but my mind was an evil twin, shaming me when I'd give in and eat a balanced meal. At times, after eating a meal and dessert, my mind convinced me to go the route of purging.

Healing first showed itself in the form of concerned friends. Listening to them, I evened out some of my eating bahaviours, though I still had a tendency towards compulsive workouts. While my mind is much gentler and more encouraging now, I still endure negative thoughts. But instead of looking in the mirror and just seeing the size of my thighs, I now see legs that are strong. I see a body that can run a half marathon and maybe more. Some runs are joy-producing, while others are downright gruelling – nevertheless, each run holds the feeling of freedom. My lungs fill and release. My legs propel me forward. Each mile, each step forward is enough."

## *Ashley

*"I was physically and emotionally wrecked."*

"I don't remember a time when I ever felt content or happy about my body. During high school, I was bullied about my weight, my appearance and, later, my intellect. Comments like "It's actually disgusting how fat she is" on top of the pressures every normal teenager faces were enough to send me down a very damaging spiral.

My focus shifted completely to my physical appearance, because that seemed to be what everyone else was focused on. I began purging. I thought if I lost heaps of weight, I wouldn't get bullied anymore and I would be skinny and happy like everyone else. That was my mentality and I stuck to it for a very long time. I would skip lunches at school, and head to the bathroom after dinner. I was physically and emotionally wrecked.

I would spend hours every single night Googling ways to lose weight fast, including diets, pills, surgeries – anything I could find. I would spend hours looking at myself in the mirror, thinking of changes I could make from head to toe. At school, I was constantly jealous of other girls and friends of mine, which caused me to become incredibly introverted. In my mind, they looked so much better than me.

University brought on a slew of more insecurities. Pool parties, beach days, and beach houses were a no-go zone for me. I didn't want to risk friends looking at me and thinking I was fat. I hated events that weren't planned weeks in advance because I needed time to prepare. My preparation was extreme dieting and exercising, and a mirror analysis most nights. I exercised for 1–2 hours a day, and I ate very few calories, often causing me to feel faint or to pass out mid-workout.

It has taken me years of therapy and self-work to get to a better mindset. I feel extremely proud of where I'm at today, but it wasn't easy. I completely cut negative people who evaluate success as having an amazing job, boyfriend, and being skinny from my circle of friends. The biggest thing I've learned is just to be kind to myself and to others. You never know what people are going through. It's so important to surround yourself with friends and family who see the good in you – both outside and in."

## BULIMIA NERVOSA

Those with bulimia will eat unusually large amounts of food for a specific period of time. Each binge eating episode continues until the person becomes overly and sometimes painfully full. During this time, bingers feel as though they can't stop eating or control how much they eat. They will binge on any type of food, but most commonly a binger will choose foods that they are trying to avoid. After the binge, bulemics will attempt to purge to compensate for the calories consumed, and to relieve their stomach discomfort. Common purges include induced vomiting, fasting, laxatives, diuretics, and enemas.

Like anorexics, bulimics will often exercise excessively to lose weight. Although symptoms are similar to anorexia, bulimics typically maintain a normal weight, rather than becoming too thin, which can make bulimia harder for others to detect. Common symptoms include:

- Feelings of being out of control with each binge episode
- Repeated purging to prevent weight gain
- Self-esteem tied to body weight and shape
- An obsessive fear of gaining weight, despite being a normal weight.

Bulimia produces numerous health risks, including an inflamed sore throat, swollen salivary glands, worn tooth enamel, tooth decay, acid reflux, irritation of the gut, severe dehydration, and hormonal disturbances. In severe cases, bulimia can also produce an imbalance in electrolytes such as sodium, potassium, and calcium, which can cause a stroke or heart attack.

## BINGE EATING DISORDER

Binge eating disorders (BED) are similar to bulimia, and are believed to be one of the most common eating disorders. For instance, typically large quantities of food are eaten in relatively short periods of time and the person feels out of control during binges. The difference is that those with BED do not restrict calories or purge by vomiting, and nor do they engage in excessive exercise. Common symptoms of BED include:

- Eating large amounts of foods quickly in secret and until uncomfortably full, despite not feeling hungry
- Feeling out of control while binging
- Feelings of shame, disgust, or guilt for eating behaviours.

Unlike anorexics, people with binge eating disorder are often overweight or obese. This may increase the risk of medical complications linked to excess weight, such as heart disease, stroke, and type 2 diabetes.

### *Casey

***"I would often feel ashamed and hide the amount of food I was eating."***

"Being overweight has influenced every single aspect of my life. The way I view myself, the choices I've made, the hobbies I did or didn't do, and, most importantly, my relationships with other people. It made me self-conscious and ashamed of my body at an unnaturally young age, and an easy target for relentless teasing and bullying in primary school. What seemed like harmless jokes ultimately laid the foundation for social anxiety and deep-rooted insecurity.

Even though I was the designated classroom clown in high school, cracking jokes and ensuring everyone around me was happy, I was really the complete opposite. Somewhere in my early teens, I learned that the more people laughed at my intentional jokes, the less likely they were to laugh at my physical appearance. As the years went on, the number on the scale kept increasing, and together with it, the hatred and disgust I felt for my body. I had trapped myself in a vicious cycle of turning to food as a source of comfort. I would stuff myself with all my favourite treats when I felt even remotely upset, which was followed closely by feelings of guilt and shame for going overboard.

During a binging episode, I would often feel ashamed and hide the amount of food I was eating by sneaking it into my bedroom when no one was watching. I was afraid of judgmental comments and overcome with feelings of shame, guilt, and disgust with myself – even while putting said food into my mouth. The next day, I would wake up to a wave of regret, determined to 'do it right' with the clean slate of the new day. But, ultimately, this cycle would repeat almost daily.

Every year, I would dread the arrival of summer and the prospect of having to wear shorts and dresses to avoid drowning in a pool of my own sweat. When I did manage to convince myself that it was too hot to be wearing jeans, I would cry in front of my bedroom mirror at the sight of my legs and the thought of having to go out in public.

Now, at 23, the relationship I have with my body is a complicated one – with ups and downs, celebrations and resentment, but, as of late, acceptance and contentment too. After years of self-loathing, the scales – no pun intended – are finally tipping to the side of truly loving myself. With the help of therapy, I have unlearned many of the unhealthy ideas that were rooted in past experiences, and instead I've finally internalised that I am deserving of the space I take up in this world, regardless of what that space may be shaped like."

## PICA

Pica is a lesser-known eating disorder that involves eating non-food substances. Although it may sound strange, those with pica will consume such things as ice, dirt, soil, sand, chalk, soap, paper, hair, cloth, wool, pebbles, cigarette ash or butts, detergent, or cornstarch. Pica can occur in teens and adults, but it is most frequently diagnosed in children, pregnant women, and those with mental disabilities. The behaviour must continue for a month or more in order to be considered pica. The health risks of pica include poisoning, parasitic infections, intestinal blockages, choking, and nutritional deficiencies, and it can be fatal depending on what is ingested.

### *What causes pica?*

Although there is no single cause, certain deficiencies such as iron or zinc may be associated with pica. An iron deficiency can be the underlying cause of pica in pregnant women, for example. People with schizophrenia, OCD, or autism may develop pica as a coping mechanism, and dieting and malnourishment can also lead to pica. In these cases, eating non-food items can help people feel full.

### *How is pica treated?*

Doctors will first treat complications from eating non-food items. If the cause is nutrient imbalances, they may prescribe vitamin or mineral supplements. A psychological evaluation may determine if OCD or another mental health condition is the root cause. Depending on the diagnosis, medications, therapy, or a combination are typical treatment options.

## RUMINATION DISORDER

Rumination disorder has recently been recognised as an eating disorder. It is a condition in which a person regurgitates food they have previously chewed and swallowed, and then either re-swallows it or spits it out. This rumination typically occurs within 30 minutes of a meal. Unlike medical conditions like reflux, it is voluntary. The disorder can develop at any stage in life from infancy to adulthood, and people with this disorder may restrict the amount of food they eat, especially in public, which can lead to weight loss.

## AVOIDANT/RESTRICTIVE FOOD INTAKE DISORDER

Avoidant/restrictive food intake disorder (ARFID) is a new name for an old disorder. The term replaces what was once known as a "feeding disorder of infancy and early childhood", a diagnosis previously reserved for children under seven years old. Although ARFID generally develops in infants and children, it can continue into adulthood. This should not be confused with picky eating in toddlers or dieters. Those with this disorder are either not interested in eating or they are repulsed by certain food smells, tastes, colours, textures, or temperatures.

Common symptoms of ARFID include:

- Avoiding or restricting food intake
- Eating habits that interfere with normal social functions, such as eating with others
- Weight loss or delayed development for age and height
- Nutrient deficiencies.

## OTHER EATING DISORDERS

In addition to those described above, there are other eating disorders, including:

- *Purging disorder.* People who control their weight through vomiting, laxatives, diuretics, or excessive exercising, but don't binge eat
- *Night eating syndrome.* Those who eat excessively at night, often waking up to binge eat
- *Orthorexia.* People who are obsessed with healthy eating to the point where it disrupts their daily lives or causes weight loss. People with orthorexia often find it difficult to eat in restaurants, and eliminate entire food groups they consider unhealthy from their diet. Charlotte, an orthorexic, explained the pain of her condition this way: "At family lunches after church on Sunday, I would spend time in the bathroom

crying over the limited menu choices, anxiously bracing myself for the horror of having to eat something that didn't meet my standard of healthy. I felt like a burden to my family and lived in guilt for how my struggles affected them."

## WHAT CAUSES EATING DISORDERS?

Eating disorders may be caused by genetics, brain biology (levels of the brain messengers serotonin and dopamine), personality traits (perfectionism, Type-A, and impulsiveness), and cultural ideals. Studies involving twins who were separated at birth and adopted by different families show some evidence that eating disorders may be hereditary. Researchers found that if one twin develops an eating disorder, the other has a 50% likelihood of developing one too.

### What parents can do

Given the rise of eating disorders in tweens and teens, how do parents know when to be concerned? Experts agree that adults should be on the lookout for abnormal behaviours, like skipping family meals and refusing to eat certain categories of food such as bread and other carbohydrates. Other warning signs are when your child suddenly loses 10 to 20 pounds, hoards food – a sign of binge eating disorder – is secretive about what they eat, obsessively counts calories, or over-exercises.

Parents should also pay close attention when teens express guilt or anxiety about food or eating, or feel unhappy with their bodies, constantly checking their weight on the bathroom scale. It's also common to see eating disorders in LGBTQ+ teens. Have a conversation with your teen about what's going on in their life and about their mental state. Eating disorders are treatable, but it's important to seek help quickly since early intervention will improve the speed of recovery and likelihood of staying free of the illness in the future.

# EATING DISORDER SELF-ASSESSMENT TEST

Do you or a loved one have an eating disorder? The following SCOFF questionnaire, developed by British researchers, is a simple, five-question screening test to assess the possible presence of an eating disorder. SCOFF is an acronym for Sick, Control, One, Fat, Food.

(Answer yes or no)

1. Do you induce vomiting because you feel uncomfortably full?
2. Do you worry you have lost control over how much you eat?
3. Have you recently lost more than one stone [approximately 6 kg or 15 pounds] over a three-month period?
4. Do you believe yourself to be fat when others say you are too thin?
5. Would you say that food dominates your life?

Results:

If you answered yes to two or more of the above questions, I suggest you make an appointment for an assessment with an eating disorder professional, such as a therapist, dietitian, or physician. A healthcare professional can determine if you suffer from anorexia nervosa, bulimia nervosa, binge eating disorder, or another type of eating disorder.

Once you've been diagnosed, a professional can recommend an appropriate treatment for you. If you didn't answer yes to two or more of the questions, but you believe you may have a problem anyway, or someone else is concerned about your eating or exercise behaviour, you may want to be evaluated because the SCOFF questionnaire does not pick up all eating disorders or disordered eating behaviours. You may still be struggling with body-image concerns, for example, or an obsession with orthorexia, in which case treatment may help you. It is also common for people with eating disorders to be in denial.

## Resources

The following organisations specialise in treating eating disorders and body image issues:

- **The Butterfly Foundation.** Butterfly's national support line 1800 ED HOPE is for people with eating disorders and anyone who has a question about them. https://butterfly.org.au/
- **Butterfly Foundation, New South Wales.** In addition to its national support line, the Butterfly Foundation also provides eating disorder recovery support groups and face-to-face low-cost counselling at Butterfly House in Crows Nest, Sydney. www.thebutterflyfoundation.org.au
- **The Butterfly Foundation, Tasmania.** The Butterfly Foundation provides face-to-face support programs as well as support groups for people experiencing body image issues as well as their carers and friends in Hobart, Tasmania. www.thebutterflyfoundation.org.au
- **The National Eating Disorder Collaboration.** This is a great resource for up-to-date information and research on eating disorders. It also provides a list of treatment services throughout Australia for inpatient, outpatient and community support programs. www.nedc.com.au
- **Health at Every Size Australia.** The Health at Every Size Australia directory provides listings of health practitioners around Australia who offer services consistent with the organisation's principles. It lists a range of services, including psychologists, nutritionists and GPs. www.haesaustralia.org.au/find-a-provider
- **Eating Disorders Victoria.** Eating Disorders Victoria is a state-based source of support, information, community education and advocacy in Victoria for people with eating disorders and their families. www.eatingdisorders.org.au
- **Eating Disorders Queensland.** Eating Disorders Queensland is a statewide, community-based, not-for-profit organisation. They promote positive body image and prevention of eating issues. Supportive therapeutic options for individuals living with eating issues and their families and friends are also offered. www.eatingdisordersqueensland.org.au
- **Eating Disorders Association South Australia (EDASA).** EDASA provides information, workshops for community professionals, and support groups for people experiencing an eating disorder and for their carers in South Australia. www.edasa.org.au

- **Women's Health Works, Western Australia.** Women's Health Works provides women with self-help groups, and a range of education, information and support for eating disorders. www.whfs.org.au
- **F.E.A.S.T.** is an international nonprofit organisation run by parents and caregivers of those suffering from eating disorders.

CHAPTER EIGHT

# YOUR SELFIE IMAGE

Like many little girls, my daughters love princesses. Their favorites are modern Disney characters, such as Moana and Ariel, along with Anna and Elsa from *Frozen*. Fortunately they are all strong female role models who don't rely on a prince to save the day, but rather seize control of their own destiny. Some of the more traditional princess stories, however, while seemingly innocent, can encourage an unhealthy preoccupation with being "the fairest of them all". To make matters worse, the evil characters are typically ugly witches or monsters.

As parents, my wife and I try to teach our girls not to have unrealistic beauty ideals, and to love themselves whether or not they fit the conventional idea of beauty. Difficult as it may be, we hope they will learn to resist, or at least question, the avalanche of media and social media influences so they can judge themselves by other criteria than how they look and behave.

## REAL VERSUS IDEAL

Teens and young women see proof of body norms everywhere. They see it at school. They see it in their sports. They see it in the media and on their phones, where they are bombarded by images of picture-perfect bodies. As active consumers, teens are bombarded by thousands of ads and Insta posts a day. What they may not realise, however, is that these airbrushed images are manipulated so dramatically they present an unattainable image of beauty. This continuous barrage of images and messages reinforces what our girls view as the ideal woman, which directly impacts their body confidence. According to a 2018 Mission Australia youth survey, body image is the fourth largest concern for teenage girls, with 30% expressing anxiety about their body image. Another survey found that looking at magazines for just 60 minutes lowers self-esteem in over 80% of girls. The truth is, the majority of photographs of women in the media are the work of makeup artists, hair and photo stylists, photoshoppers, and professional lighting. But that's not where the magic ends. Digital retouchers make thighs thinner, bellies flatter, and skin flawless. Our smartphones can do a bit of digital retouching using filters and by adjusting the light and tone too. Photos are often so altered that the women are unrecognisable. When you add the splashy headlines that are often disparaging of real women, it's no wonder that girls crave that perfect photoshopped look.

Actress Kate Winslet, who starred in *Titanic* when she was 21, was outraged when she saw how her legs had been slimmed down in a cover photo for *GQ* magazine. She responded by saying "The retouching is excessive... Practically every photo you see in a magazine has been digitally altered in this way." After that, she took legal steps to protect her real image in an ad she did for the cosmetic company L'Oreal by putting a clause in her contract that said images must be free of any additional editing. "I do think we have a responsibility to the younger generation of women," Winslet said in an interview with E! News. She added that being in the spotlight gave her an opportunity to promote a positive body image message to young girls around the world.

Surveys confirm the need for girls and women to see models and celebrities in a more realistic light. In its Pretty as a Picture survey, advertising think tank Credos asked young women to compare four different images of the same model that had been digitally altered to change her shape. The majority (76%) preferred either the natural or lightly retouched images to the heavily airbrushed ones. Similarly, the Dove Global Beauty and Confidence Report found that 69% of women and 65% of girls believe media and advertising set an unrealistic standard of beauty that most women can never achieve.

One of the contributors to female body image concerns, according to the American Psychological Society (APA), is the manufacture of sexy clothing in child and teen sizes. The APA Task Force Report on the Sexualization of Girls, which was first released in 2007, noted that some retail stores now sell intimate apparel for tweens and teens, including sexy lingerie, camisoles and lacy panties – items that were once only available in women's shops like Victoria's Secret. Kohl's, the national retail chain, offers a juniors' thong, for example. Similarly, the report goes on to say Halloween costumes made especially for girls and young women frequently emphasise physical attractiveness in beauty queens, princesses, and sexy cheerleaders. Among the few female villain costumes, sexual eroticism was emphasised, as in Sexy Devil.

The toy and cosmetics industries have followed this trend by marketing their products to younger and younger girls. Toy shops sell a Girls Ultimate Spa and Perfume Kit "… perfect for spa parties, sleepovers, and rainy days"; the Body Shop has lip glosses intended for teens, and fruity lip glosses for preteens; Claire's, an accessory store in thousands of malls, sells lip gloss and perfume to young girls. Barbie has perfumes called Free Spirit, Summer Fun, and Super Model.

The APA researchers conclude that the sexualisation of girls and women has negative consequences in a variety of domains, including cognitive functioning, physical and mental health, sexuality, and attitudes and beliefs. The messaging from the media, particularly companies like Disney, has traditionally been of the male character being the beast, whereas girls are always portrayed as delicate and pretty with unrealistic body ideals. Fortunately, this has changed recently with strong female characters like Moana and Princess Merida in Brave, who buck the trend of the helpless and hapless princess.

**What parents can do**

Although it's impossible to shield your teen from these idealised versions of beauty, parents can teach their teens to be media and marketing literate. Encourage your daughters to start thinking more critically when viewing pictures of celebrities and models. Have conversations with them about the ways media images are manipulated, and emphasise that they rarely represent real, inclusive, and diverse beauty. Help them understand that they shouldn't compare the way they look to the fake images they see. Here are some suggestions for how to do this:

- **Use real examples.** When you're watching TV together, pause shows and commercials to talk about the messages that are being conveyed. Look at magazines together and discuss the unrealistic images you see in ads and photo shoots
- **Talk about marketing.** Discuss the tactics advertisers use to sell products. Help your daughter spot underlying messages about how a product will make her more attractive
- **Have conversations about unhealthy body images.** Discuss the harsh realities that underweight models face. Tell your teen about the drastic and unhealthy measures many take to obtain these body types like the ones I wrote about in the previous chapter, and the toll it takes on their health.

Conversations like these will help your daughters develop a healthy body image.

## SOCIAL MEDIA MARKETING

Currently, I am the NSW State Chairperson of Training Junior Plastic Surgeons; I also sit on the national education board for the Australian Society of Plastic Surgeons (ASPS). So for me, the use of social media ties into my passion for teaching and mentoring students, colleagues and patients alike. There isn't a day that passes that I don't get a question about how to perform procedures from colleagues all around the world, which is thoroughly rewarding. I try to keep this perspective in mind when creating social media content. However, as informative as I make my posts, the ones that garner the most attention, reach, and engagement are the ones that show the most dramatic cosmetic changes in patients, not the educational posts.

Medical advertising ethics change over time. Starting in 1847, advertising was forbidden by the American Medical Association's Code of Ethics, until the Federal Trade Commission (FTC) declared the stipulation a violation of restraint of trade and, therefore, illegal. Practice websites, online before-and-after photographs, and plastic surgery reality television shows have travelled a similar arc. Consequently, I believe plastic surgeons must maintain ethical standards while adjusting them to meet changing norms – in other words, set standards for professionalism. Professionalism transcends ethics and, in plastic surgery, consists largely of abiding by what resonates with physicians as human beings, and the image they want to portray to their audience as well as the rule of law.

In Australia, we have very strict and transparent rules regarding medical advertising guidelines established by the Therapeutic Goods Administration (TGA). A unique rule we have in Australia, that other Western countries do not, is that it is illegal to have any patient testimonial on an advertising platform that you control. This means no testimonials on our websites, and the review tab on Facebook has to be turned off. This includes turning off comments on all Instagram and social media posts. A short summary of the Medical Board's set of guidelines that all medical practitioners must abide by is below.

The requirements for advertising and marketing therapeutic goods must:

- Be conducted in a manner that promotes the quality use of the product
- Be socially responsible
- Not mislead, deceive the consumer or trivialise surgery
- Be accurate, balanced and substantiated
- Only make claims that are consistent with the advertised goods' indication or intended purpose

- Have the relevant mandatory statements, including health warnings where applicable. Health warnings must be displayed or communicated before any purchase is initiated, including from social media. In social media, the mandatory statements and health warnings must be visible at all times, and not within collapsed information as that does not meet the requirement of being prominently displayed or communicated. For example, after every social media post that I upload I must add *"Any surgical or invasive procedure carries risks. Before proceeding, you should seek a second opinion from an appropriately qualified health practitioner."*
- Not claim that a product can diagnose, treat or cure a serious condition without prior permission or approval from the TGA
- Not contain testimonials or endorsements which breach the Code due to their potential to create unrealistic expectations of beneficial treatment. This includes re-sharing stories or posts from patients that are recommendations or positive statements about the cosmetic surgery and/or interacting with the review, such as liking or otherwise responding to a patient's social media post.
- Presents the risks and recovery process of cosmetic surgery accurately
- All medical practitioners advertising cosmetic surgery must include clear and unambiguous information about their qualifications and type of medical registration
- Cosmetic surgery advertising must not use terms (including in taglines, hashtags and similar) that advertise the medical practitioner or the medical practitioner's abilities in a manner that may be misleading or create unrealistic expectations. Examples of inappropriate terms include 'magic hands', 'sculptor', 'god', 'queen', 'world's best', 'world renowned'
- Cosmetic surgery advertising must not offer incentives, gifts, discounts or inducements that would encourage people to have cosmetic surgery.
- Single images must not be used in cosmetic surgery advertising when the use of the image is likely to give the impression that it represents the

outcome of a surgery as this can mislead the public, idealise cosmetic surgery and/or increase unreasonable expectations.

- Images of people aged under 18 years of age must not be used in advertising of cosmetic surgery
- 'Before and after' images must be as similar as possible in content, lighting, camera angle, background, framing and exposure, posture, clothing and make up.
- Images and/or videos must not idealise or sexualise cosmetic surgery through the use of sexualised images, contain nudity, use emotive emojis to cover body parts or use lifestyle shots of patients

## SOCIAL MEDIA AND SELF-ESTEEM

In 2021, a whistleblower who worked at Facebook (now Meta) revealed internal memos and research from the company showing that Instagram, which is owned by Facebook and a platform frequently used by teens, is harmful to girls' body image and well-being. The social media monolith swept those findings under the rug, says the former employee, and continued to conduct business as usual. Facebook's policy of pursuing profits regardless of documented harm has sparked comparisons to Big Tobacco, which famously denied the health risks of smoking cigarettes. This news does not come as a surprise to anyone who follows social media, as studies consistently show that the more often teens use Instagram and other social media, the worse their overall well-being, self-esteem, life satisfaction, mood, and body image.

Similarly, girls feel anxious and suffer emotionally from the attention they get from posting suggestive videos on TikTok, according to therapists. TikTok has grown in popularity amongst tweens and teens, reaching one billion users last year. The company's algorithm calculates whether viewers show strong interest in a particular type of content, measured by whether they finish watching videos. Its recommendation engine then chooses videos to send to those viewers.

Platforms like Instagram, YouTube and Twitter work differently, serving content to users based on search terms and friend connections, so developing a sizable following – and going viral on those sites – can take longer. A TikTok company fact sheet says "content that is overtly sexually suggestive may not be eligible for recommendation." Their spokeswoman also said content from users who state they are under 16 isn't eligible for promotion via the recommendation engine, nor would it appear in search results.

The problem, however, is that teens are known to lie about their age when creating social media accounts. Users must be 13 to have a TikTok account, and it is company policy to suspend the accounts of kids the safety team believes to be underage. Nevertheless, many underaged users slip through the cracks, and teens are reportedly suffering emotional distress from oversharing explicit content. According to a program director from Newport Academy, a mental health and rehab center for teens based in Atlanta, Georgia, 60% of the girls treated in its 2021 outpatient program have posted sexually inappropriate videos on TikTok.

In my own practice, I've seen patients who unfavourably compare themselves to the people they see online. And with an increasing number of influencers filing up people's feeds, it's easy to imagine how impressionable tweens and teens feel unworthy by comparison. Kim Kardashian and the Jenner sisters, for example, have a combined 600 million followers – far more than the entire population of Australia. Today's average teen spends about six hours per day on social media, according to a report by Common Sense Media, and what they are seeing online can determine how they view themselves. A staggering 62% of teens report dissatisfaction with how they look on social media, according to the American Academy of Facial Plastic Surgery.

The role of influencers cannot be understated in the cosmetic surgical industry, but fortunately Australia, through the TGA, has some very strict rules regarding this, in that it is illegal to provide surgical and medical services in exchange for promotions. This is considered inducement and not a favourable behaviour when establishing a doctor-patient relationship. I receive about one message per month from influencers who want free surgery in exchange for promoting my business on their various channels. One influencer was taken aback and shocked when my staff charged her for a consultation. Fortunately, she went elsewhere, and I did see her posts promoting her eventual surgeon. Another influencer sent me her usual rates for different post types, for example an Insta story cost less than a feed post. She wanted to barter the number and quality of her posts in exchange for surgery. Shocking, I know.

The TGA in 2022 took extraordinary steps to outline the rules and behaviour of influencers when related to medical products. In short, the TGA allows influencers to give testimonials for products, but only if they receive nothing in return. This lack of freebies for influencers means most of them don't bother to endorse, as the advertising code applies to all medicines, medical devices, vitamins and supplements, and general health products. The TGA stipulates that if you are an influencer who is involved with a therapeutic goods company, and you have been paid or given a product by the company to promote its goods, you should consider the following:

- Any post about a therapeutic product that you make may be considered advertising. If it is, you have an obligation to comply with the advertising requirements for therapeutic goods
- Any comments you make about your personal experience with therapeutic products or services amounts to a testimonial. Testimonials are not permitted by those involved in the production, sale, supply or marketing of the goods. Your social media posts may have an impact on your followers' beliefs, attitudes, preferences and behaviours. Your comments about therapeutic goods can influence consumers' choices. Therapeutic goods should be chosen on the basis of clinical need, not through the persuasion of influencers

- Understand what the approved purpose of the product is, and do not advertise for any other purpose, whatever your experience with the product.

I mention this so you know what's going on behind the social media curtain, and judge what you see online with a more critical eye. Is the source honest and reliable? Is there a quid pro quo arrangement between influencer and advertiser? Are you being manipulated by the images you are seeing? Seeing is not always believing, so keep all this in mind when you are envy scrolling.

## DEPRESSION AND SOCIAL MEDIA

Researchers are just beginning to establish a link between depression and social media. While they have not actually discovered a cause-and-effect relationship between them, they have found that social media use can be associated with an intensification of the symptoms of depression, including a decrease in social activity and an increase in loneliness. According to a survey of 14–24 year olds conducted by the Royal Society for Public Health, use of Snapchat, Facebook, Twitter, and Instagram have all led to increased feelings of depression, anxiety, poor body image and loneliness.

In a 2016 study of social media and body image for women, researcher Markia Tiggemann and colleagues also concluded that "frequent social media use has been related to more body image concerns and eating disorders". Further evidence shows that the more social media you consume, the greater its impact on your mental health. Another study, published in *Computers in Human Behavior*, found that the use of multiple social media sites is more strongly associated with depression than the amount of time spent online. According to this study, people who used more than seven social media platforms had more than three times the risk of depression than those who used two or fewer sites.

Additionally, the liberal use of filters to change one's selfie snap has contributed to this negative self-image. Social media has introduced new clinical challenges, including what is known as Snapchat dysmorphia. Filters may lead to an altered sense of appearance in reality, and as a plastic surgeon I need to be wary of this when consulting with patients. Dr. Dariush Nikkhah, a London-based plastic surgeon who has visited my clinic, said younger patients may feel pressured to attain the perfect breast shape or perfect nose due to social media exposure, which prompts them to undergo unnecessary procedures. In his 2016 article that appeared in *Aesthetic Surgery Journal*, he wrote:

> *"If you think that you or your child may have Snapchat dysmorphia, consider the following: do you look only at what others are posting, or are you taking, filtering, and uploading selfies? Do you constantly check your posts for the number of likes. Do you measure your appearance based on how many likes you received? For many who post on social media, it's all about the numbers. Self-worth gets tied up with likes, comments, and views. Are you following close friends and family, or a bunch of celebrities and influencers? Research suggests that who you compare yourself to is key to your self-image, and that peer feedback can be addictive for those whose self-esteem depends on social media affirmation."*

Jasmine Fardouly, a researcher at Macquarie University in Sydney, Australia, says that teens who compare their appearance to those on Instagram, TikTok, Snapchat, or whatever platform they're on, often judge themselves unfavourably. The reason for this, Fardouly explains, is that people present a one-sided version of themselves and their lives online. If it's a close friend or family member, you know them well enough to judge whether or not they are showing only the best bits, but if it's an acquaintance or famous

YouTuber, you won't have enough information to properly judge the veracity of the post.

This finding was echoed by Candice E. Walker and colleagues in their paper 'Effects of social media use on desire for cosmetic surgery among young women', published in a 2019 issue of *Current Psychology*. The research suggests that young women's desire for cosmetic surgery is increased by viewing images of females who have undergone cosmetic enhancements, especially if the viewer is less satisfied with their appearance.

"Fitspiration" influencers are another group of popular posters who may make you judge your body more harshly. They are typically beautiful, well-toned people exercising or showing off athletic or yoga moves. I have seen many such athletes as patients, and I am often surprised how different they look in real life compared to their social media posts – at times unrecognisable. Amy Slater, an associate professor at the University of West England, Bristol, published a study in which 160 female undergraduates viewed either #fitspo, self compassion quotes, or a combination of both on Instagram. Those who viewed only #fitspo scored lower on self-compassion, but those who saw the compassionate quotes such as "You're perfect just the way you are" were kinder to themselves and felt better about their bodies. Those who looked at both #fitspo and self-compassion quotes were able to overcome their negative body image – a testament to the power of positive messaging.

Young people who are continuously taking and posting selfies frequently need reassurance that they look good, but even with a large number of likes, that affirmation is fleeting, and only lasts as long as it takes to post another selfie. If any of this rings true for you, and you find it impossible to put down your phone, make sure to engage in activities that don't have anything to do with appearance or comparisons. Think seriously about whom you follow, and if you find yourself facing an endless stream of appearance-focused photos the next time you scroll, try switching to humour or cute animal pictures instead. I realise that giving up social media altogether is too big of an ask, but finding inspiring or humorous memes and images on your Instagram or TikTok feed might just help you remember there's more to life than how you look.

## INDIRECT COMMUNICATION

In an article published by the Child Mind Institute, when teens are not doing their homework – and even when they are – they're online and on their phones, texting, sharing, trolling and scrolling on their devices. Prior to Instagram and TikTok, teens were likely to communicate by chatting on the phone, or in person hanging out at the mall. Whilst these activities may seem similarly aimless, experts say hanging out allows teens to exercise social skills, and that teens today are missing out on these developmentally important real-time interactions by hiding behind their screens.

"As a species we are very highly attuned to reading social cues," Catherine Steiner-Adair, EdD, a clinical psychologist and author of *The Big Disconnect*, was quoted saying. "There's no question kids are missing out on very critical social skills. In a way, texting and online communicating – it's not like it creates a nonverbal learning disability, but it puts everybody in a nonverbal disabled context, where body language, facial expression, and even the smallest kinds of vocal reactions are rendered invisible."

## LOWERING THE RISKS

Learning how to make friends is a major part of growing up, and friendship requires a certain amount of risk-taking. When a friendship is conducted online and through texts, kids aren't hearing or seeing the effect that their words might have on the other person. Because the conversation isn't happening in real time, each party can take longer to consider a response. No wonder kids eschew talking on the phone, finding it too intense. It requires more direct communication, and if you aren't used to that it may well feel scary.

If kids aren't getting enough practice relating to people and having their needs met in person, many of them will grow up to be adults who are anxious about our most basic form of communication – talking. And the problem will only get worse as they begin navigating romantic relationships and social interactions at work.

## *Grace, 17

*"The cuter or sexier it is, the more LIKES you get."*

"After you start posting for a while, you learn what type of pictures get the most LIKES. The cuter or sexier it is, the more LIKES you get. Some people post 20 times a day, and most people add a filter to their selfies. You just kind of start doing those things without realising it. Over time, it can become overwhelming, if that's the only thing that I'm focusing on. I feel like the older I get, the more insecure I am about my face and body. And it doesn't help to look at other beautiful selfies. Now I try to be really mindful whenever I'm going to post something; I make sure that it's coming from a good place with the right intentions."

## What parents can do

Whilst unplugging from devices is not realistic, there are ways that parents can curate social media feeds so their girls feel happier in their own skin – or at least stop feeling worse. Talk to your daughters about social media use. This is the best way to protect your child from risks and ensure their internet safety. Topics to discuss should include:

- How they treat other people and how they want to be treated online. Encourage your teen to make only positive comments

- The risks involved in using social media. Make sure your child understands the danger of sexting or being tagged in an embarrassing photo taken at a party
- How to navigate posting risks. For example, if your daughter posts an identifiable selfie, she can reduce risk by not including any other personal information
- What to do if people ask for personal information
- How to deal with ghosting – when someone suddenly stops texting and responding – catfishing – having a false persona online – and other online relationship issues.

## CYBERBULLYING

One of the most troubling aspects of social media is cyberbullying. Hiding behind a screen makes it easier for teens to say what they would never dream of saying to face-to-face. This is especially true of girls who don't like to disagree with each other in real life, but if they bully it's usually done with mean-spirited gossip and social exclusion.

Typical teen cyberbullying involves abusive texts and emails, hurtful messages, embarrassing images or videos, intimidation, exclusion, or nasty online gossip. It can happen to anyone, even people considered popular at school, and causes the victims to withdraw and feel shame, guilt, fear, loneliness, and depression. Because teens spend so much time online, it can be hard for them to escape cyberbullying. The nasty messages spread like wildfire, and are difficult to delete. When the bullies are anonymous, it's harder to put a stop to it. Here are some more sobering facts about cyberbullying:

- One in five young Australians has reported being cyberbullied
- Most cyberbullying occurs amongst teens from 14–17
- Approximately 50% of victims know their cyberbully, who is usually another student at the same school

- Girls are more likely to be victims
- Girls are more likely to spread rumours
- Boys are more likely to post hurtful or embarrassing pictures and videos
- Cyberbullies are generally the same age as their victim
- Approximately half of the victims met their cyberbully online, and did not actually know them.

## CYBERBULLYING WARNING SIGNS

Many kids who are cyberbullied don't tell adults what's going on. They're afraid their parents will overreact, and make the situation worse or separate them from those they consider friends. The following are some warning signs that a tween or teen may be the target of cyberbullying:

- Skips school or is reluctant to go
- Falls behind in homework
- Stops using devices
- Becomes withdrawn, distressed, anxious
- Has lowered self-esteem and confidence
- Becomes aggressive and begins to bully others
- Has trouble sleeping
- Becomes moody, depressed, angry or frustrated
- Isolates themself from peers and family
- Has suicidal thoughts – this should be treated by a mental health specialist.

### *Charlotte's Story

*"I have learned that things stay on the internet forever and can come back to haunt you later in life."*

"I posted a photo of myself on Instagram with the caption 'Life is good'. A bunch of people, including a boy I previously was hanging out with, attacked this post with really mean and rude comments about me. I was so upset that I privately texted the girl who seemed to be leading these comments asking her why she was writing these hurtful things. She replied by saying 'it's a joke and we are just having fun.' She then continued to write more mean things about me, and she threatened me saying that she would hurt me and live stream it for other people to watch.

"I was scared, and devastated when students from my grade, whom I thought were my friends, commented about how funny she was and how annoying I was. People from other high schools whom I didn't know even chimed in! I felt attacked and all alone. My close friends tried to comfort me privately, but no one had the courage to actually defend me on social media. I had this horrible sinking feeling of everyone hating me and talking about me behind my back. Some of my sympathetic friends even wrote to me that they would 'hang themselves' if people were writing these kinds of things about them. I was so confused and sad that I decided the right thing to do was tell my mum and my family. My mum reached out to my school advisor, who reminded us that my school has a code of conduct policy that includes a cyberbullying section that all students sign.

"I have thought about this a lot, and realise now how important it is to be careful about what you put online. I have learned that things stay on the Internet forever, and can come back to haunt you later in life. The Internet is definitely not the right place to let your emotions and angry feelings towards a person or situation out. I was very hurt by this experience.

"Recently, the girl who wrote all those things about me and I got together. She apologised to me for the things she had posted, and we decided that moving forward we would both do our best to look out for each other and only spread kindness out on social media. To anyone going through this, remember you are not alone. Don't be afraid to ask for help and to share your story. It will get better, I promise."

**What parents can do**

If your daughter is showing any of the above warning signs, tell her you are concerned and that you want to help. Let her know she can come to you for help if she sees anything inappropriate, upsetting or dangerous online. If she won't open up to you, recruit other people to talk to her, such as a trusted teacher, guidance counsellor, or relative. The following are some other tips for combatting cyberbullies:

- Discuss rules for online safety and Internet use. Ask your teens to contribute to establishing the rules, as this way they'll be more inclined to follow them
- Tell your children not to respond to cyberbullying threats or comments, but not to delete any of the messages. Instead, print out all the messages, including the email addresses or social media handles of the cyberbully. You may need these as proof of cyberbullying if you take further action
- Be supportive and understanding. Let them know they are not to blame for being bullied. Find out how long the bullying has been going on, and assure them that you'll work together to find a solution
- Don't tell them to shrug it off or just deal with it. The emotional pain of being bullied is very real and can have long-lasting effects. Don't take a kids will be kids attitude
- Don't threaten to take away your teen's phone or computer. This only forces them to be more secretive if they are having a problem
- Get the school involved if the cyberbully is a classmate. Schools should take cyberbullying seriously. Most do, and staff can take action to stop the bully and help protect your child during the day.
- If there are threats of physical violence, get law enforcement involved.

## PORNOGRAPHY

If you're a teenager reading this, chances are you've already watched porn. You probably watched on one of your devices, or maybe you happened to see some pictures on your friend's phone or laptop that one time. Whatever the case is for you, research shows approximately 40% of 13-year-old girls and 67% of 13-year-old boys have seen at least one pornographic image online in the past year. By the age of 18, over 60% of girls and over 90% of boys have seen porn in some form or other.

Whatever you and your family believe in terms of sexual mores, I want to address the impact porn can have on a young girl's body image. If you decide to watch Pornhub, keep in mind that pornography isn't real: it's entertainment and it's an aphrodisiac. I can tell you as a plastic surgeon that most porn actresses have had some kind of cosmetic enhancements on their breasts, lips, and other body parts. Be careful not to form unrealistic expectations of how people actually look based on what you see on sex videos. The popularity of labioplasty procedures has been linked to the rise in access to pornography – and this goes for the men, as well. The average man is not as generously endowed as the male porn stars. The danger in watching a lot of porn while you are a tween or teen is that you are still forming your personal and sexual identity. You don't want to feel badly about your own body because you don't look like a porn star.

### *Meaghan's story

***"Whilst it may feel like everybody's doing it… it isn't normal to send nude images of yourself."***

"A few years ago, when I was 15, I was tricked into sending an image of myself with no clothes on to someone who I thought was a boy I'd been chatting with online, but it was actually a girl in my year group. He or she asked me 'Can you send a photo of yourself?' I answered no in the beginning. But being a teenager and having the phone constantly in my hand, the pressure just didn't stop. 'He' just kept asking,'Why are you saying no? Everybody does it. You're just being frigid.'

The pressure did eventually get to me, and I just thought okay, this is the normal thing, and if this is going to get someone to like me, why shouldn't I do it? About an hour afterwards, I received a Snapchat picture of the girl saying 'Ha ha, I got you!' I went to school the next day hoping that, even though she had played a horrible trick on me, she wouldn't be so nasty as to send it around. But as soon as I walked into school, I felt like a zoo animal; everybody was just crowding round me laughing and talking about it. I was classed as a prostitute, as sort of a stripper because everybody had seen my body. I thought I was worthless.

I actually told the school police about what happened. The girl who tricked me didn't get into trouble, and I was made out to be the one at fault. Whilst it may feel like everybody's doing it, I bet you they're not. It isn't normal to send nude images of yourself. If you send an embarrassing image, talk to someone. Don't keep it to yourself. A problem shared is a problem halved."

### What parents can do

Talking to your daughters about pornography can be uncomfortable, but open and honest discussions lead to healthier future relationships. Here are some important things you could talk about:

- **Porn is a business.** Explain that, like Hollywood movies, people in the porn industry have sex to make money. As with many jobs, some people willingly choose to take part in making pornography, whilst others do it because they need the money
- **Porn stars are actors.** Young people may think that pornography shows them what sex and bodies should look like. You can explain that the people you see in porn videos and films are actors. There is a

director who tells them what to do, and they have to look like they're having a great time – even when the sex is not pleasurable

- **Porn and relationships.** Teens who look at pornography regularly may develop unhealthy views about gender roles, sex, and sexual performance. This can make it harder for them to develop respectful and enjoyable sexual relationships. Talk to your teen about fulfilling relationships that are about emotional closeness and trust, as well as mutually enjoyable sex. Hardcore pornography can make violent sex and disrespectful relationships seem normal
- **Nonconsensual porn.** Nonconsensual pornography can take many forms, but all cases have one thing in common – someone has shared a private image of the victim without their consent. Tell your daughter that she should never post compromising sexts, even if they are to a boyfriend. Sexting also has some unexpected legal consequences that parents and many teens are simply not aware of, including the fact that over 90% of all sexting images will end up on other social media sites. The current federal law makes it illegal to take, share, keep and distribute images of a sexual nature by phone or online, including someone who is sending images of themselves, if the person involved is under 18.

**And tell your sons not to ask, pressure or threaten girls about their unwillingness or refusal to send images of themselves.**

## Resources

- **eSafetyWomen.** eSafetyWomen is designed to empower Australian women to take control of their online experiences. The eSafetyWomen resources aim to help women manage technology risks and abuse by giving them the tools they need to be confident when online. www.esafety.gov.au/women
- **Youth Law Australia** is a community legal service that is dedicated to helping young people in Australia find a legal solution to their problems. https://yla.org.au
- **eSafety** is Australia's independent regulator for online safety. They educate Australians about online safety risks and help to remove harmful content. https://www.esafety.gov.au
- If you have been bullied or witnessed others being bullied and need help, you can contact **Kids Help Line** (1800 55 1800), which is a free and confidential telephone counselling service for 5–25 year olds in Australia. http://www.kidshelp.com.au
- **Lifeline** (13 11 14) is a free and confidential service staffed by trained telephone counsellors. www.lifeline.org.au
- **The Australian Human Rights Commission** (1300 656 419) has a dedicated service that investigates complaints of discrimination, harassment and bullying. www.humanrights.gov.au/complaints_information/index.html.

CHAPTER NINE

# #YOUTOO?

When I first started writing this book, the Australian government was in the throes of a sex scandal: Brittany Higgins, a former political adviser to the ruling Liberal Party, had accused a male colleague of raping her in Parliament House. Her story triggered a flood of other women who came forward with their own experiences of alleged sexual assault and harassment in the Australian government. News stories like these make it clear that sexual harassment, abuse, and assault is pervasive, and is something I want my daughters to be aware of as they grow up. It's our job as parents to teach our sons to respect women, and to teach our daughters how to protect themselves at school, work, and life in general.

## WHAT IS SEXUAL HARASSMENT?

As our children develop sexually, they become curious about their bodies, their gender, and sex. By the time they reach puberty, this sexual awakening is not always pleasant. Boys may begin to talk disparagingly about girls' bodies and make unwanted advances. Whilst some of this is a natural part of development born out of curiosity, sexual harassment has nothing to do with mutual attraction or consensual behaviour. It's unwanted or unwelcome sexual conduct that is offensive, humiliating, or intimidating. Here are some examples of sexual harassment that can happen in primary, middle, and high school:

- Unwanted physical contact, such as touching, bumping, grabbing, or patting
- Sexually insulting remarks
- Bragging about sexual prowess to others
- Intimidating behaviour, such as demeaning nicknames, homophobic name-calling, cat calls, rating appearance, or wolf whistles
- Slut-shaming graffiti written on restroom walls, lockers, or desks
- Being stalked or followed by another student.

The more sexual harassment girls experience, the more likely they are to feel emotional distress, depression, embarrassment, poor self-esteem, suffer from substance abuse, and have suicidal thoughts. Their attitudes about their bodies take a nosedive, with many girls disliking how they look and developing eating disorders. Despite this, girls rarely report incidents to teachers or parents and, in most cases, they don't tell the harassers to stop – largely due to a concern about social consequences.

A 2019 survey of adolescents conducted by Plan International found more than 60% of teen girls worry about retaliation if they confront or report their harasser. More than half of girls worry that people won't like them if they say something, or that people will think they are trying to cause trouble or just being emotional. Half think they won't be believed.

Most say they try to forget about or ignore the harassment, chalking it up to just part of life they have to deal with as a girl. The problem with trying to ignore sexual harassment, however, is that it doesn't work. Research on the most effective ways to cope with stressful events shows that seeking social support and confronting the source of the distress are far more effective than trying to downplay or ignore the problem.

## TIKTOK TACKLES HARASSMENT

There are myriad reasons teens may harass sexually: it makes them feel powerful; they want to appear sexually mature; it helps them bond with peers. Sexual bragging or put-downs are also a way to wrestle with insecurity and low self-esteem.

A recent TikTok video that has been liked by almost half a million viewers encourages girls to record themselves putting one finger down for every time they were sent unsolicited sex pics, begged for nudes, catcalled, repeatedly asked out after already saying no, or forced to do something sexual when they didn't want to. By calling attention to how common sexual harassment is for teenage girls, the *Put a finger down: sexual harassment edition video* is the 2021 TikTok version of the #MeToo movement that began in 2006 to raise awareness of sexual abuse. It is a way to help teens cope with an age-old problem using a medium they are comfortable with. Seeing all the posts lets these girls know that they are not alone.

## *Makailah

***"Every day guys make comments about girls' bodies."***

"Every day guys make comments about girls' bodies, especially at at my school, and especially to me, because I'm built different. I remember one time somebody asked me 'How much?' like I was a sexworker while I was in school. I didn't say anything about it. I wanted to, but it's just really embarrassing to go to an administrator and say 'People are looking at me this way.' That was in 10th grade, so last year. It was somebody I knew. It was at lunch. It just gave me the chills. When stuff like that happens to me, I'm not sure how to react. Sometimes I'll just go along with the crowd, because I don't want to seem like I'm a party pooper. It just really made me feel uncomfortable. Even before I was insecure about that, but now I feel really insecure. Now I feel like I have to cover myself up and hide myself. Teachers don't really say anything about it, and students don't really say anything about it. My friends talk about this all the time. But sometimes we're not really sure how to feel. We haven't really been taught about what we should say, and what we should do. At my school, we don't have resources. We don't have anything regarding consent. I really try my best when I see things like that happening to other girls. There was a time I interned at this community centre, and there was a kid guy who was kind of cornering a girl. I didn't like that he was doing that. I knew it was making her feel unsafe. I told him, 'You can't do that. That's not okay.'"

### What parents can do

It is vital to prepare your daughters for some of the disturbing situations they may encounter at school. Parents can do this by giving their children age-appropriate lessons on sexuality and personal boundaries. Try to instil a sense of confidence in them in the face of their harassers. Teach them to make eye contact, and to be assertive. Help them to build self-esteem. Here are more ways parents can start talking about sexual harassment and how to combat it:

- **Define the problem.** Start by asking your teen to define sexual harassment by giving them examples of what it means. Make it clear that even if what's said is intended as a joke, it can still be hurtful and offensive
- **Speak up.** Tell your daughter that silence won't make the problem go away. Encourage her to either confront the harasser, perhaps with a friend in tow for support, or talk to a teacher or school counsellor. Consider rehearsing the conversation with your teen so she feels more comfortable
- **Esteem-building activities.** Encourage your daughter to get involved in activities that build confidence but don't involve sexual attention or approval from peers, such as sports, art, music, science, or service to others.

## STALKING

The Australian Bureau of Statistics found one in six or 1.6 million women has been stalked at least once since the age of 15. Stalking is when someone repeatedly contacts you, follows you, sends you things, or threatens you. Although anyone can be stalked, it often occurs either as part of an abusive dating relationship or after the relationship has ended. Examples of stalking behaviour include:

- Showing up at the same places or events
- Following or lurking near your home
- Watching from a distance
- Repeatedly driving by the victim's home or workplace
- Taking photos without permission
- Calling or texting repeatedly
- Sending unwanted emails or texts (cyberstalking)
- Sending letters or leaving notes
- Stealing or damaging property
- Spreading rumours.

### *Bella

*"I hid in my house as he was knocking on my door."*

"My heart goes out to anyone affected by stalking. I've been stalked twice. One was a work colleague whom I dated for a short time in my early twenties, and then decided to end it. He would buy me gifts, hang around my office, cry, coerce me back into being with him, and even threaten to kill himself. He had been considered a star at that company. I left to go back to school and was relieved by the timing of that, which helped remove me physically from the situation.

Interestingly, he reached out and contacted me a couple of years ago. Because his email address used his surname in plural, I thought he was happily married and it was safe to respond the once, out of that ever-present female politeness thing. I discovered he was no longer working due to health reasons, and lived with his parents. The pattern immediately reappeared. His first email was full of flattery, and I responded politely with a very broad update (we were in different countries, so it felt safe to do so), and said I would not be renewing ongoing contact. I then got an abusive email about all of my shortcomings. I blocked him.

The other incident was when I saw a younger man as a fling, which for him turned into perceived love. He lived in Canberra, and I was in Sydney. I communicated, but I didn't want to continue seeing him, and he sent gifts to try and convince me otherwise because, as he saw it, I was his "the one". Then one day he rang to say he was on his way from Canberra to see me – yes, I made the mistake of answering the phone, but he was my flatmate's brother and I was trying to handle it all politely and not burn bridges with my flatmate. I, of course, insisted he did not come, and actually hid as he was knocking on the door – he had driven all the way up from Canberra. I felt awful about myself – that maybe somehow I was being the horrible one to him. I was also clear that I did not want to develop a relationship with him as his extreme ardor in such a short space of time, and really little substance between us, and the deafness to my feedback, were confirmation for me. I guess both times I was lucky it did not escalate into one of those truly nightmarish stories. It still impacts me, because these incidents have made me wary of men showing me too much affection and attention in the early stages."

## What parents can do

Because stalking can escalate into physical violence or sexual assault, it's important to take precautions to ensure your daughter's safety. Be as vigilant as you can, and never hesitate to contact the police if you believe your child is in danger. When it comes to stalking or any unwanted attention, here are some things you and your teen can do:

- **Identify safe spots.** If your daughter is being followed, it's important she knows where to go to stay safe. If she drives, make sure she knows where your local police station is and how to get there. Tell her never to hesitate to call 000 if she feels she is in danger
- **Help your teens vary their routines.** Walking the dog or going for a run at the same time every day makes it easier for the stalker to know where

she will be and when. Likewise, the person may know your daughter's favorite hangouts, and even where her friends live. Tell her to change habits, so a stalker won't know where to find her

- **Go out in groups.** Being alone, especially at night, is risky for someone who is being stalked. For this reason, your daughter should get a walking buddy, or always plan to go out in groups. This includes going to the shops, running errands, and studying at the library. Make sure you have your daughter's buddy's number.
- **Use phone safety etiquette.** Posting on social media about where they are or what they are doing gives a stalker way too much information. Even if she has blocked the person from her accounts, stalkers can still find out the information from posts by friends and acquaintances.
- **Don't respond to messages.** It's never a good idea to respond to someone who is stalking, cyberbullying, or harassing. Even just telling them to stop could be enough attention to keep the stalker engaged.
- **Keep you informed.** While your daughter may baulk at this request, it's important that she keep you informed of her whereabouts at all times. This way, if something happens, you will know approximately where she is and whom she is with should you need to find her.
- **Trust your gut.** Most teens tend to downplay things or assume that they are overreacting, even when their gut is telling them otherwise. Talk to your teen about the importance of trusting their instincts. If they feel like something is wrong, it likely is.
- **Let school officials know.** Even though being stalked may be embarrassing for your teen, it's important that other people know what's going on. School officials can be an extra pair of eyes on the lookout for anything out of the ordinary, and will alert the police if necessary.

## DATING ABUSE

The stats on teen dating abuse in Australia are the stuff of nightmares. Surveys show that 33% of teenagers report knowing a friend or peer who has been hit, punched, kicked, slapped, choked or physically hurt by a partner. Alarmingly, Australian research also indicates that teens aged 14–19 are up to four times more likely to experience physical or sexual violence than older women. Reports of sexual assault reached a six-year high in 2017, according to the ABS. Equally disturbing is that many young women don't even realise they are in abusive relationships.

The problem of teen dating abuse, which includes controlling behaviour, verbal insults, emotional manipulation, and sexual coercion as well as physical assaults, has reached frightening proportions. Like the other high-risk behaviours in this book, teenaged girls who have been in abusive relationships have an increased risk of substance abuse, eating disorders, and even suicide. Warning signals usually start appearing when a girl is in a toxic relationship, but many parents – and teachers – frequently miss the signs that their daughter could be dating someone dangerous.

### *Rachel's story

*"I truly believed all the fights were my fault."*

"I met my boyfriend online when I was just 13. He was 18 and lived across the country, so we texted and talked on the phone for months before meeting in person. When I was a sophomore in high school, he moved to my hometown so we could be together. I had always been super-involved at school – honour roll, student council, sports. After he moved here, he felt my activities were taking me away from him. He would pick fights with my family, and say that I had to choose between the two. If I didn't choose him, he said I didn't really love him. Before I got counselling, I truly believed all the fights were my fault. He convinced me that he was perfect and it was me who needed to change. I'd say 'Okay, I want to change. I love you. I can be better. Give me another chance.'

The emotional abuse continued, and things went from bad to unbearable after we started living together. I had gotten into a good university, but I decided to move in with him instead. My parents were furious and said they would support me as much as they could, but I was basically on my own. I got a job at a daycare centre and he managed a pizza place. Things were good for about a month, but then he'd tell me 'You promised to change, but you haven't and you're ruining my life.' Then he'd hit me. The first time he backhanded me he gave me a fat lip. He was so worried someone would notice the bruises and report him, he'd make me call in sick until I healed. He also said it was my job to satisfy him every day, and if I didn't he'd find another girl.

Six months later, he called me at work to ask where I put the laundry cart. When I couldn't remember, he told me I was irresponsible and threatened to come to work. I took care of babies, so I said I had a family emergency and went home. When I got home, he used my body as a punching bag. That was the last straw for me – I left him after that."

## MINAH STEIN

Here's what American university student Minah Stein wrote for MTV News about why she became an advocate for young women who are victims of sexual assault:

> *"I didn't set out to become an activist. Activism found me four years ago at the age of 12, when my friends started to date. One couple became legendary at our school, but not in a good way. One day I'd see them walking hand-in-hand, the next day they would be screaming at each other. Broken up? Madly in love? No one could keep track.*

*Teens I talk to now tell me that every school has 'this couple.' Everyone seemed to just shrug the behaviour off, but I didn't get it. Was this normal? Is this what I had to look forward to when I started dating? I did some research, and what I learned shocked me: unhealthy relationships start early and can last a lifetime.*

*I decided to make a video with facts about domestic and teen dating violence. Other kids volunteered to help me out. We showed the video at school club meetings throughout our county, and found that most students hadn't realised that unhealthy relationships could spin out of control and create perpetual patterns of abuse. Guys were particularly shocked to learn that they could become victims of dating violence too. The video made students think about what they would accept from a dating partner – something they hadn't been aware they should consider. This work gave me confidence in my own voice. I learned that anyone – including teens – can effect change, and realising this made me want to do even more.*

*Around this time I heard a radio program talking about sexual assault. I couldn't stop thinking about what I had learned from that episode, including that about 1 in 5 girls will be sexually assaulted while in college, as will 1 in 16 boys, but that roughly 80% don't report the assault. What really haunted me, however, was the fact that this problem doesn't begin in college – it begins in elementary and secondary schools.*

*These weren't just statistics: they were people – students, just like my friends and me. At first I was scared, but then I became angry. Why weren't more teachers or administrators talking to us about sexual assault? If these statistics represented a disease that could be inoculated against, schools would mandate that every student be vaccinated for our own protection. Sexual assault is an epidemic in our secondary schools and our universities, and yet there is still more that needs to be done. Sexual assault education should be a mandatory subject in every elementary, middle, and high school across our country and at our universities.*

*Until it is though, I'm on a mission to teach students the facts about what constitutes consent, how to stay safe, and what their Title IX rights are. In 2014 I formed EMPOWERU, a community action program that aims to do just this. And I joined the advisory board of Stop Sexual Assault in Schools. In April 2015, with the help of my EMPOWERU Ambassadors, I held a countywide pledge drive at area high schools to encourage students to take a pledge against sexual assault. Over 200 students took the pledge.*

*During this campaign, I was shocked by the range of students' responses. Many were put off by having to confront the reality of sexual assault. Perhaps they were scared or didn't believe it could happen to them. On the flip side, a few e-mailed me to say they or a friend had survived a sexual assault, and thanked me for my work. Both of these reactions affirmed that doing this work with my high school peers is necessary.*

*I wanted to do more, but quickly found that doing so was an uphill battle. It took eight months of meetings with school officials and local sexual assault experts to screen the documentary* It Happened Here *at each of the high schools in my county. Eventually, however, I succeeded and played a key role in helping over 1,500 kids learn about sexual assault… My work is far from done. I won't rest until students, younger and older, are educated about the very real dangers of sexual assault and about their own Title IX rights so they are prepared to deal with this problem."*

*NOTE: Title IX is a civil rights law in the United States that prohibits sex-based discrimination in any school or other education program that receives federal money. Every American educational institution receiving federal funding is required to have a Title IX coordinator whom victims can contact to report sex discrimination, sexual harassment or violence. Australia does not have a similar law.*

## What parents can do

Tell your daughters that a healthy relationship is one where a partner doesn't try to change or control them. A relationship should consist of patience, trust, kindness, love, and understanding. Above all, love does not hurt. Look out for the following signs that your daughter may be in an abusive relationship:

- She used to have more friends than she does now
- She used to be outgoing and involved with family and school activities
- She frequently cries or is sad
- If her boyfriend texts her, she has to reply immediately
- He is jealous if she looks at or speaks casually with another boy
- He dictates her choice of friends, hairstyle, clothes, or makeup
- He is aggressive and quick to anger
- She makes excuses for his poor behaviour or says it's her fault
- He calls her demeaning names, then laughs and tells her he was only kidding
- She frequently has to apologise or explain herself to her boyfriend
- She has bruises she can't explain.

As much as you may want to step in and physically remove her from the situation, you need to let her recognise that the relationship is unhealthy. Unless she is at risk of harm, it's best to allow her to make the decision on her own terms. If you push her too soon, your plans may backfire and she may feel even more committed to her boyfriend.

## DATE-RAPE DRUGS

Sadly, young women who are single must watch out for another potential danger in the form of date-rape drugs, which include alcohol and some medications. These substances make it easier for someone to rape or sexually assault someone: a famous example of this is comedian Bill Cosby, who was convicted in 2018 of putting Quaaludes in women's drinks so they would have sex with him. The person who's been drugged may become confused, have trouble defending themselves, pass out, or not be able to remember what happened later. Also, date-rape doesn't always happen on a date. An attacker could be someone you just met, or someone you've known for a while.

## COMMON TYPES OF DATE-RAPE DRUGS

- *GHB (gamma-hydroxybutyric acid).* This depressant has many nicknames: easy lay, liquid X, liquid ecstasy, liquid E, grievous bodily harm, Gib, G-riffic, scoop, soap, salty water, organic Quaalude, and fantasy. Doctors sometimes prescribe it to treat a sleep disorder called narcolepsy.
- *Rohypnol (flunitrazepam).* This is a strong benzodiazepine (a class of tranquilisers) also known as Mexican Valium, circles, roofies, la rocha, roche, R2, rope, and forget-me pill. It's not legally available in the United States, but in other countries doctors sometimes use it as anaesthesia before surgery.
- *Ketamine.* This is a dissociative drug that makes you feel detached from reality. Its nicknames include Special K, vitamin K, and cat Valium. Doctors and veterinarians use it as anaesthesia. Researchers are also studying it for people who have severe depression.
- *Alcohol.* Many attackers use one of the aforementioned drugs along with alcohol. It can boost the medicine's effects, but alcohol by itself can also keep you from defending yourself, knowing what's happening to you, or remembering it later.

## DATE-RAPE DRUG EFFECTS

- GHB can make you sleepy, forgetful, or weak. It can also cause seizures, a slow heartbeat, slow breathing, and a coma. The effects start in 15–30 minutes and last 3–6 hours.
- Rohypnol relaxes you. In high doses, it can make you lose control of your muscles, produce amnesia, loss of inhibitions, and loss of consciousness. Its effects usually start within 30 minutes and peak about two hours after you take it. As little as 1 milligram can affect you for 8–12 hours.
- Ketamine may make you hallucinate or feel woozy. It can also cause an upset stomach, vomiting, high blood pressure, changes in your heart rate, seizures, or a coma. It usually takes effect within 30 minutes and lasts an hour or two, but you may be affected for a day or more.
- Alcohol may make you feel more relaxed, chatty, and confident. As you drink more, your emotions become unstable, and you lose control of your body. Drinking too much can also put you in a coma. Alcohol usually enters your brain within a few minutes, and is particularly dangerous for teens whose brain is not yet fully developed.

## HOW TO AVOID DATE-RAPE DRUGS

A few tips can help keep you stay safe when going to a bar or party:

- Pour your own drinks. Avoid open containers like punch bowls that could be spiked. Don't accept drinks from other people
- Keep control of your drink at all times. Carry it yourself, even if you have to take it to the bathroom with you
- Don't drink anything that tastes strange
- Stick with your friends. Ask them for help if you suddenly feel sleepy.

## WHAT TO DO IF YOU THINK YOU'VE BEEN DRUGGED AND RAPED

If you suspect you've been drugged and assaulted, call the police or have a friend take you to the emergency room. The authorities will collect evidence, so try not to pee, bathe, wash your hands, or change clothes before you go to hospital. Tell the doctors or people treating you what happened. Ask for a urine test as soon as possible, so drugs can be detected before your body flushes them out.

No matter how much you drank or what drugs you took, sexual assault is never your fault. It's common to go through a range of emotions afterwards. Talk to someone you trust or call 1800 737 732, open 24-hours a day, seven days a week.

## POLICE CONTACTS

*Australian Capital Territory*

AFP Police
www.police.act.gov.au/connect-us

*New South Wales*

NSW Police Sexual Assault Reporting Options (SARO)
www.police.nsw.gov.au/community_issues/adult_sexual_assault

*Northern Territory*

NT Police Sex Crimes Division
Ph: 08 8922 3617
www.pfes.nt.gov.au/Contact-us.aspx

*Queensland*

Reporting to Qld Police – Information
www.police.qld.gov.au/programs/adultassault/report/#reportAssau…

Alternative reporting options
www.police.qld.gov.au/programs/adultassault/altReportOpt.htm

### *South Australia*

SA Police Sexual Crime Investigations
Ph: 08 8172 5555 (business hours only)
www.police.sa.gov.au/contact-us/key-contacts

### *Tasmania*

Tasmania Police Contact
www.police.tas.gov.au/contact-us

### *Victoria*

Local Sexual Offences and Child Abuse Investigation Team (SOCIT) locations and phone numbers
www.police.vic.gov.au/content.asp?Document_ID=36448

### *Western Australia*

WA Police Sexual Assault Squad
Phone: 08 9428 1600
Email: SexAssaultSquadSMAIL@police.wa.gov.au
www.police.wa.gov.au/Your-Safety/Sexual-assault

**Resources**

- For more information about sexual assault services in Australia, visit Rape and Domestic Violence Services, Australia. www.rape-dvservices.org.au
- Relationships Australia (1300 364 277)
  Support groups and counselling on relationships, and for abusive and abused partners. www.relationships.com.au

CHAPTER TEN

# TATTOOS, PIERCINGS, AND OTHER BODY ADORNMENTS

The trend in body adornments is still going strong in Australia, with the number of young people getting tattooed or pierced continuing to rise. Three in five, or 60% of Australians, now have more than one tattoo. Although ear piercings are the most common, one in five teens has had other parts of their body pierced, including the tongue, lips, and navel. For teenagers, the popularity of body art comes from a desire to make a fashion statement, wanting to be like peers, expressing identity and individuality, or rebelling against parents.

Whatever your feelings are about body art and jewellery, parents should try not to overreact if their teen tells them they want to get inked or pierced. If you hate the idea of tattoos or body-piercings, your child may be more willing to listen when you discuss your opinions calmly without forcing your values onto them. It is perfectly reasonable to inform them of the laws regarding minors, or say "I don't like the idea of you getting a tattoo at 16, because you may decide you don't like it in five years' time." Here are some things you should know before you or your child becomes a human canvas:

## TATTOOS

A tattoo is a permanent kind of body art. A design is made by puncturing the skin with needles, and injecting ink, dyes, and pigments into the deep layer of the skin. Tattoos used to be done manually – that is, the tattoo artist would puncture the skin with a needle and inject the ink by hand, but though this process is still used in some parts of the world, professional tattoo artists now use tattoo machines. A tattoo machine powers the needles up and down as ink is deposited in the skin.

### *What to do before you tattoo*

If you're thinking of getting a tattoo, remember that removal is difficult, expensive, and may not completely take off the tat. Tattoo removal lasers never remove the tattoo back to virginal skin, in fact they leave the skin with a faint outline of the tattoo, which actually looks worse than having it there in the first place. The only way to remove a tattoo completely is with surgery, but you are swapping one problem with another – a scar or need for a skin graft.

Make sure you have had all your immunisations, especially hepatitis B and tetanus shots, and if you have heart disease, allergies, diabetes, skin problems like eczema or psoriasis, a weakened immune system, or a bleeding condition, talk to your doctor beforehand. Also, people who are prone to keloids, which are raised scars, should probably not get a tattoo. Even though tattoos are fashionable at the moment, having one done in a place that you can't cover with clothing, such as your face or neck, could hurt your chances of getting a job or advancing your career in certain professions.

### *What are the laws for tattoos and branding minors?*

If you're under 16, you cannot get a tattoo or be branded in Australia, but if you're between the ages of 16 and 18, you can get both as long as you have written permission from a parent. In Victoria, South Australia, Tasmania and Queensland, it's a criminal offence for a tattooist to work on someone under 18, and in the Australian Capital Territory and New South Wales, teenagers under 18 years need their parents' permission for tattoos.

Professional studios typically take pride in their cleanliness, but here are some things to ask the manager or tattoo artist:

- Does the tattoo studio only use single-use needles and sterilise all equipment with an autoclave that employs steam, pressure, and heat for sterilisation? Needles and other equipment must be removed from sealed, sterile containers
- Do they use one-time ink cartridges that are disposed of after each customer?

- Is the tattoo artist a licenced practitioner? The tattoo artist should be able to provide you with references
- Does the tattoo studio follow standard procedures for dealing with blood and other body fluids to help prevent the spread of HIV, hepatitis B, and other serious blood infections?

If the studio looks unclean, or something looks out of the ordinary, or you feel in any way uncomfortable, find another studio.

### *What's the procedure like?*

Here's what to expect:

- The tattoo artist will wash their hands with antibacterial soap and water and wear clean, fresh gloves and possibly a surgical mask
- The area on your body getting tattooed should be washed with soap, and shaved if necessary. The artist will draw or stencil the design on your skin
- The area is cleaned again with alcohol or an antiseptic, and a thin layer of ointment such as petroleum jelly is applied
- Using a tattoo machine with sterile needles attached, the tattoo artist will begin drawing an outline of the tattoo. The artist may change needles, depending on the design and desired effect, but all needles should be single-use or sterilised
- Any blood or fluid is wiped away with a sterile, disposable gauze or cloth
- When finished, the area, now sporting a finished tattoo, is cleaned once again and a bandage applied.

### *Does it hurt?*

Getting a tattoo hurts, but the level of pain can vary, depending on your pain threshold, what body part you are tattooing, the size and number of needles being used, and the artist's style – some are quick, some work more slowly, and some are more gentle than others. Anything over a bony prominence hurts more than over muscle. It can feel like scratching, burning, stinging, or tingling. Some people feel sharp pains, while others may describe the feeling as dull.

### *Taking care of a tattoo*

Follow all of the instructions the studio gives you for aftercare, and to make sure you heal properly:

- Keep a bandage on the area for 24 hours
- After 24 hours, remove the bandage and keep the tattoo open to air
- Avoid touching the tattooed area, and don't pick at any scabs that may form
- Avoid clothes that may stick to the healing tattoo
- Wash the tattoo with soap and warm water – don't use alcohol or peroxide – then use a soft towel to dry the tattoo. Just pat it dry and do not rub it
- Apply antibiotic ointment, thick skin cream, or vitamin E oil to the tattoo two to three times a day for a week. Don't use petroleum jelly
- Do not let the tattoo soak in water. Showers are fine but avoid swimming and baths until the tattoo is fully healed
- Keep your tattoo out of the sun until it's fully healed
- Lifelong maintenance of your tattoos with sun protection to avoid them fading.

A tattoo usually takes about two weeks to heal. Even after it's fully healed, wear sunscreen with a minimum SPF of 30, as this not only protects your skin, but can help keep the tattoo from fading.

### *What are the risks?*

Some people have allergic reactions to tattoo ink, causing itching, bumps, and rashes that may occur days, weeks, or longer after the tattoo was done. Tattoos can also make eczema, psoriasis, or other skin conditions flare up.

Never tattoo yourself or have a friend do it for you. Skin infections caused by bacteria, viruses, or fungi can occur if the skin is not cleaned properly, or the ink and needles are contaminated. Sharing needles, ink, or other equipment without sterilisation increases your risk of getting HIV, hepatitis

B, or hepatitis C. Call your doctor right away if you have bleeding, increased pain, or signs of infection.

### *Tattoo removal*

Many people love their tattoos and keep them forever, but others decide at some point that they really don't want that snake on their arm or their ex's name on their chest. If this is the case, laser treatment is the best option for removal, but be warned the laser never removes the tattoo back to normal skin. The success of the laser also depends on your skin type, how big and complex the design is, and the types and ink colours that were used. The laser sends short zaps of light through the top layers of your skin, with energy aimed at specific pigments in the tattoo. Those zapped pigments are then removed by the scavenger cells or phagocytes from your body's immune system. Other less common ways to remove tattoos include dermabrasion, chemical peels, and surgery.

It can take several months of treatments, and results are not guaranteed. Treatment can cause darkening or lightening of the skin, and scarring. Removal can also be expensive. I frequently see patients who have tried laser removal with varying results, but you need to then decide whether you want to swap the tattoo for a scar or skin graft. Which is worse?

## BRANDING

Branding involves burning the skin with hot or cold instruments to produce a permanent design. While the results may be similar to a tattoo, branding is much riskier. Unlike tattoos that can be removed with laser surgery, or pierced holes that can heal, branding is permanent. It's a painful process that should only be done by professionals who are trained in handling sterilised equipment in a sanitary environment.

## BODY PIERCING

Body piercing is exactly what it sounds like – a piercing or puncture made on the face or the body by a needle. After that, a piece of jewellery is inserted in the hole. Commonly pierced body parts include the ears, nose, navel, lip, cheek, tongue, and nipples. After a piercing has healed, some people expand the size of the hole, typically in the earlobe, to wear certain types of jewellery such as plugs or flesh tunnels. Stretching should be done in small increments to reduce the chance of scarring or damage to the piercing.

### *Take precautions*

Like tattoos, make sure you've had all your immunisations, especially hepatitis B and tetanus shots, before getting pierced. If you have a medical problem, such as congenital heart disease, allergies, diabetes, a weakened immune system, or a bleeding condition, talk to your doctor first. And if you plan to get a tongue or mouth piercing, make sure your teeth and gums are healthy. Also, if you are prone to keloids you should probably not get body piercings.

### *What are the laws regarding minors?*

In some parts of Australia (including Victoria), it's illegal for a piercer to perform intimate piercing on anyone under the age of 18 years, whether or not consent has been given. This includes piercing of the genitalia or nipples. In the Australian Capital Territory, Northern Territory and Queensland, teenagers under 18 can get body piercings as long as they can make a sound and reasonable judgement. In Western Australia, teenagers under 18 years can get body piercings with a parent's permission.

### *What to look for*

Like tattoo studios, it's a good idea to do some investigative work about a shop's procedures to find out whether it provides a clean and safe environment. Every shop should have an autoclave sterilising machine, and keep sterilised instruments in sealed packets until they are used. The shop also should follow procedures for the proper handling and disposal of waste such as needles or gauze with blood on them. Make sure you're not allergic to any metals, and choose jewellery, including backs or studs, made from metals that are less likely to cause reactions, such as surgical stainless steel, solid gold (not gold-filled or gold-plated), niobium, or titanium.

### *What is the procedure like?*

Here's what to expect when getting a body part pierced:

- Body piercers should wash their hands with antibacterial soap and water and wear clean, fresh gloves
- The area to be pierced (except for the tongue) is cleaned with alcohol or another antiseptic
- The piercer will remove needles and equipment from sterile containers
- Your skin is punctured with a very sharp, single-use needle
- The piece of jewellery, which has already been sterilised, is inserted
- The body piercer disposes of the needle in a special container so there is no risk of the needle or blood coming into contact with anyone else
- You will get instructions on how to care for your new piercing, and what to do if there is a problem.

### *What are the risks?*

It's normal to have mild swelling and tenderness at the site of the piercing. Swelling may be significant in the case of a tongue piercing. Serious problems can occur if you try to pierce yourself or have a friend do it for you. Make sure it's done by a professional in a safe and sterile environment. Common problems related to body piercing include pain, infection, bleeding, scarring and keloids, and allergic reaction to jewellery.

Infections can range from skin or cartilage redness, swelling, tenderness, and pus, to more serious infections like toxic shock syndrome, blood infections, tetanus, and hepatitis. Tongue swelling and jewellery in the mouth may block the airway, causing serious breathing problems. There is also a chance that jewellery in the nose may be swallowed or inhaled into the lungs.

### *Piercing care*

Depending on the body part being pierced, healing time may be a few weeks to several months. Make sure to take good care of the pierced area afterwards – don't pick or tug at it, and keep it clean with water and mild soap, not alcohol or hydrogen peroxide. Always wash your hands before touching a piercing. If you have a mouth piercing, use an alcohol-free, antibacterial mouthwash or other recommended oral cleanser. Call your doctor right away if you have bleeding, increased pain, or any signs of infection.

## BODY PAINTING

An alternative to permanent tattoos is body painting. Indian body painting, called mehndi, has the beauty and cachet of the real thing, without the pain or permanence. Mehndi is the 5,000-year-old art of body painting using henna. In India, mehndi is done for celebrations and auspicious occasions such as weddings.

### *How is it done?*

The henna paste is squeezed onto the skin with an applicator that looks like a small pastry tube. The dark squiggles and scrolls are left on the skin to allow the design to set, usually overnight. When the dried paste is flaked away, it leaves a stained skin pattern of tints that can range from orange to deep red. Application can take minutes for a small anklet pattern to hours for the full works on palms and feet.

### *What are the risks?*

Henna paint is a herbal compound that rarely causes allergic reactions. The depth of colour that can be achieved depends on skin type and the length of time the henna paste is allowed to set.

### *How long does it last?*

Mehndi designs fade with washing and rubbing. They can last from one to three weeks if protected with a coat of oil.

# FINAL THOUGHTS

One of the takeaway messages to my daughters and to the readers of this book is "love thyself." Not in a narcissistic way, but in a way that makes you proud, self-assured, and accepting of your flaws. The kindness that you show yourself sets the bar for how others will treat you. To those girls and young women who struggle with body image – it gets better. As I've said throughout this book, beauty is about confidence, not an unrealistic, idealised version of perfection. Confidence and resilience often come with age.

And while it's fine to want to make physical improvements if there is something that is causing you distress, as we get older the goal is to spend less time thinking about and obsessing over our appearance. Channel that energy instead into forging healthy, loving relationships with friends and family, and discovering ways that you can help others and improve the world at large.

Beauty is also about kindness, joy, and making others feel comfortable when you are with them.

It's important to surround yourself with people who love you (faults and all), and want only the best for you. Pay attention to how the people around you make you feel. Do they lift you up or bring you down? Are they constantly judging you, or do they accept you for who you are? The people you spend time with can influence your thoughts and attitudes about yourself more than you think. So if you feel bad about yourself or the way you look after spending time with someone, rethink the relationship. Conversely, be an attentive, non-judgemental friend who listens.

# ACKNOWLEDGEMENTS

This book and the adventures I have gone through was never going to be a self promotional book that most plastic surgeons write. It was always about my core belief of helping my daughters navigate their way through self-image and body development, and helping parents and tweens navigate through these challenging times. I would like to think I achieved that.

As I sit down about to send the final manuscript to the publisher for layout and printing I can't help but think that writing acknowledgements feels like writing your own eulogy. A way of thanking all of those that helped you get you to where you are and reflecting on a journey. In a way writing this book has been an awakening. What started as an innocent letter to my daughters has turned out to be a journey of enlightenment. It reminds me of the 90s movie starring Tom Cruise *Jerry Maguire*. In the film, Tom Cruise's character has a moment of clarity in a hotel room where he decides as a sports agent he needs to focus on harbouring relationships with fewer athletes and care more about their wellbeing and growth. His life goes into a tailspin as he loses clients, his fiancée and close relationships, but ultimately at the end he nurtures true friendships, love and contentment and purpose at work. Ultimate happiness. Something he hadn't expected, an unintended but pleasant consequence.

Whilst my journey hasn't had the obstacles his did, what started as a letter to my eldest daughter turned out to be more than a simple letter. The end product is a book that, even if no one reads it, has created a special bond between me and my three daughters.

Like Jerry Maguire, I had the idea to write this book in a whimsical moment in our kitchen (his was in a hotel room) one summer's morning. I was unconsciously incompetent on the processes involved in writing a book. They do say ignorance is bliss for a reason. I am more sports, science and maths than art and literature. My high school friends Chico and Briony will attest to that.

Not long after my initial thought, I recall sitting in a pub on the Isle of Wight in England on Christmas Eve after watching a classic British pantomime, talking to my sister in law and her friend about my ideas and this book, not knowing what lay ahead for me. The self doubt, writer's block, the loss of focus and, of course, the pandemic. Despite all of this, I had a task and I owed it to my daughters and myself to finish it.

As the launch date for the book nears and word has gotten out about the book I have been inundated with kind words by patients and people messaging me looking forward to reading the book. One such patient mentioned this at the end of a consult and I was nervous about the release. She reassured me that everyone that puts their ego on the line will face the imposter syndrome and you have to accept it and own it. You may recall one of my patients in the case study with Gigantomastia, she emailed me last month telling me not only has she finished her research in medical science but she is now a medical student on her own path to becoming a doctor. My daughters will go to the same high school as her which closes the circle somewhat in my mind.

So many people are to thank for this book, first and foremost are my family. Literally and figuratively I couldn't have done it without them. First shout out will always go to my wife Jodie. Her support and sacrificing her career for our family has allowed me the luxury of not only working on this book, but also pursuing my career and my dreams. She has all of the traits that I lack, and she ingrains these beliefs into our three daughters along the way educating me. The most important one being, above all else be kind and nice. Being a surgeon's partner is not easy – the brutal hours during residence are now replaced with countless hours not only running a private practice but also all of the governance work I do for the teaching societies and colleges along with my guest speaking roles at international conferences. If you have read this far in the book Jodie, thank you.

My daughters, Rosie, Evie and Tessa. All uniquely special in their own way. They won't know how lucky they are to have each other. I sat all three down the other day and said, 'You know whichever out of you three plays golf will be my favourite'. They huddled together after my speech and Rosie the eldest and spokesperson for the trio said "Daddy, just because it's your dream doesn't mean it's ours". Mike drop.

My mum and dad left war-torn Iran post revolution in 1983 for Australia, like most migrants sacrificing all to give me and my younger brother (who was one month old) a chance of a better life. My parents, like me and my wife, are opposites but each has taught my brother and I valuable lessons which have led to where I am now. My mother, a preschool teacher, has taught me the importance of cherishing friendships and family and prioritising these above all; my father taught me the power of hard work and perseverance. Sadly his and my dreams of me becoming a professional athlete vanished when at the age 17 it dawned on both of us that I didn't have "It". Better a small hurt now then than a wasted life chasing an unreachable goal. I would like to think my second choice career as a surgeon is a worthy substitute.

My mum taught me emotional intelligence and my dad taught me about grit before it was a fashionable topics on "TED Talks."

I would like to thank Jaqui Lane, The Book Adviser, for helping me take my scribble and turning it into a book. I was never going to beg a publishing house to take on my book, but I didn't know where start. Our chance encounter was a moment of serendipity. I was playing golf and I was walking down the 12th fairway with a member called Peter Ritchie. Pete is retired but he brought McDonald's to Australia. He was writing a book about how McDonald's grew in Australia. We started talking about each other's books and how Jaqui was helping him publish his project. The connection was made. Even more convenient was that Jaqui lived three blocks from my house in Sydney, making catch up sessions easy over a flat white at our local cafe. Jaqui has not only been my book advisor but as launch date nears she has been my therapist. She assures me, everyone goes through the same self doubt.

I would also like to thank Jodie Gould, a native of New York and accomplished author who I engaged through a random network of connection starting with my dear friend Eben Harrell who is an editor for *Harvard Business Review*. Her help with research and interviewing patients has been invaluable and there is no way this book would have started without her guidance and gentle nudging. Jodie was my ChatGPT, a fountain of knowledge that helped create the backbone for this book, establish a process for writing and a mission statement.

# ABOUT THE AUTHOR

As a plastic surgeon, I work with women and girls who hate something about their bodies or their appearance. It got me thinking about my conflicting roles as a father of daughters and a plastic surgeon, and how I could teach my daughters to be confident in their own skin.

I felt compelled to write this book to encourage teens to examine the media images and social pressures that blur the lines between ideal and real. I want them to know the facts about their bodies and what's "normal", and what to expect should they decide to fix something they dislike about their appearance.

I want to empower young women to reclaim their self-esteem, to know that how they look is not their fault, that beauty is about confidence, not perfection.

I also wanted to give parents, family and friends a tool to help raise body-positive girls.

**NORMAL** begins with a letter to my daughters. The title comes from comments many of my patients share with me: "Thank you, Dr. Moradi, for making me feel normal."

**Why me? If not me, who?**

I am a specialist plastic surgeon based in Sydney and hold dual post graduate qualifications as a Member of the Royal College of Surgeons of England and Fellow of the Royal Australasian College of Surgeons in Plastic and Reconstructive Surgery. I completed my training in Plastic Surgery in Sydney and have also worked in specialist surgical units in England and

Europe. I have published in peer-reviewed articles and have passion for clinical leadership and education.

Outside my private practice, I am a consultant Plastic Surgeon at Prince of Wales Hospital, the Royal Hospital for Women's and Sydney Children's Hospitals where I predominantly perform microsurgical reconstruction for breast and facial cancer patients.

Contact me: https://drmoradi.com.au